THE DOPAMINE RESET - 21 DAY DETOX

The Ultimate Guide to Reset Your Dopamine Levels, Rid Yourself of Social Media Addiction, Remove Instant Gratification, and Rewire Your Distracted Brain

LEO BLACK

© **Copyright 2024 - All rights reserved.**

The content contained within this book may not be reproduced, duplicated or transmitted without direct written permission from the author or the publisher.

Under no circumstances will any blame or legal responsibility be held against the publisher, or author, for any damages, reparation, or monetary loss due to the information contained within this book, either directly or indirectly.

Legal Notice:

This book is copyright protected. It is only for personal use. You cannot amend, distribute, sell, use, quote or paraphrase any part, or the content within this book, without the consent of the author or publisher.

Disclaimer Notice:

Please note the information contained within this document is for educational and entertainment purposes only. All effort has been executed to present accurate, up to date, reliable, complete information. No warranties of any kind are declared or implied. Readers acknowledge that the author is not engaged in the rendering of legal, financial, medical or professional advice. The content within this book has been derived from various sources. Please consult a licensed professional before attempting any techniques outlined in this book.

By reading this document, the reader agrees that under no circumstances is the author responsible for any losses, direct or indirect, that are incurred as a result of the use of the information contained within this document, including, but not limited to, errors, omissions, or inaccuracies.

TABLE OF CONTENTS

Introduction 1

Chapter 1 4

Understanding Dopamine and Its Influence 4

    The Definition and Function of Dopamine 5

        The Connection Between Dopamine and Addictive Behaviors 5

        How Dopamine Functions 6

    How Dopamine Affects Motivation and Pleasure 6

    The Brain's Reward System Explained 9

        How the Brain's Reward System Works 9

        The Role of Dopamine in Reinforcing the Reward System 10

    Key Takeaways of Dopamine and Its Influence 10

Chapter 2 12

Recognizing Your Addictive Behaviors 12

    Symptoms of Dopamine Dependence 13

    Assessing Technology Addiction 15

        Screen Time Analysis 15

        Behavioral Patterns 15

        Impact on Well-Being 16

        Detox Necessity 16

    Unhealthy Eating Patterns 17

    Substance Abuse and Other Addictive Behaviors 19

Ways to Navigate Addiction 20

Do You Recognize Your Addictive Behaviors? 21

Chapter 3 .... **22**

Preparing for Your 21-Day Detox **22**

Creating a Supportive Environment 23

    Organizing Your Space 23

    Creating a Schedule 23

    Practicing Mindful Consumption 24

Detox Essentials and Supplies 25

Setting Realistic Goals and Expectations 27

Involving Friends and Family for Support 29

    Building a Support Network 30

    Accountability Partners 30

    Seeking Professional Help 31

    Communication Strategies 31

    Celebrating Progress 32

How to Prepare for Your Dopamine Reset 32

Chapter 4 .... **34**

Week 1—Eliminating Overstimulating Activities **34**

Techniques for Unplugging From Technology 34

    Implementing Digital Detox Practices 35

    Creating Technology-Free Zones 36

    Setting Specific Time Limits for Social Media and Device Usage 36

Healthy Food Alternatives 37

Replacing Harmful Activities With Productive Ones 39

Key Takeaways for the First Week of Your Dopamine Reset 41

Chapter 5 43

Week 2—Recalibrating Your Reward System 43

Understanding and Navigating Withdrawal Symptoms 44

How to Handle Your Withdrawal Symptoms 44

Building Resilience Through Discomfort 47

Embracing Discomfort 47

Shifting Your Mindset 47

Practicing Self-Compassion 48

Developing Endurance 49

Practicing Gratitude and Mindfulness 49

Engaging in Creative and Non-Stimulatory Hobbies 51

Exploring Creative Outlets 51

Engaging Intentionally 52

Finding Balance 52

Unearthing Personal Fulfillment 53

Key Takeaways for Week 2: Resetting Your Reward System 54

Chapter 6 55

Week 3—Establishing New Habits 55

Tracking Progress and Acknowledging Milestones 56

Creating Routines That Support Well-Being 58

Morning and Evening Rituals 58

Practice Physical Activity Regularly 58

Reflective Journaling 59

Building Social Connections and Community Involvement 59

The Beauty of Social Connections 61

- Key Takeaways for Week 3 of Your Dopamine Reset 62

Chapter 7 63

Enhancing Focus and Mental Clarity 63

- Meditation and Mindfulness Techniques 63
  - Implementing Regular Meditation Practices 64
  - Mindfulness in Daily Activities 64
  - Breathing Techniques for Calmness 65
- Cognitive Exercises and Brain Games 66
  - Puzzles and Memory Challenges 66
  - Critical Thinking Exercises 67
  - Implementation Tips 67
- Cognitive Behavioral Therapy for Addiction 68
  - How CBT Works 70
- The Impact of Sleep on Focus 71
- How to Gain Mental Clarity and Focus During a Detox 73

Chapter 8 75

Scientific Insights Into Dopamine and Addiction 75

- The Neuroscience Dopamine Regulation 76
- The Role of Genetics in Addiction 77
  - Environmental Factors Influencing Dopamine 77
- Future Directions in Dopamine Research 79
- The Path to Overcoming Addiction 83
  - Resources for Overcoming Digital Addiction 83
  - Resources for Overcoming Food Addiction 84
  - Resources for Overcoming Substance Addiction 84
  - Focusing on Mental Health 85

Key Insights Into the Science Behind Dopamine and Addiction 85

Chapter 9 87

Maintaining Balance Post-Detox 87

Monitoring and Adjusting Post-Detox Habits 88

Establishing a Routine for Check-Ins 88

Utilizing Habit-Tracking Tools 88

Seeking Continuous Help From Accountability Partners 89

Consistency in Monitoring 90

Establishing Long-Term Plans 91

Staying Motivated and Rewarding Yourself 91

Continual Self-Assessment and Reflections 92

Dealing With Setbacks and Maintaining Vigilance 94

Use Mistakes as Learning Curves 94

Implementing Coping Strategies 95

Staying Present 95

Building Resilience 96

Learning From Life's Challenges 96

Long-Term Strategies for Balanced Living 96

Prioritizing Self-Care 97

Exploring New Activities 97

Establishing Boundaries 98

Seeking Professional Support 99

Recapping Maintenance Strategies for Post-Detox Success 99

Chapter 10 101

Success Stories and Real-Life Applications 101

Personal Accounts of Successful Detox Experiences 102

    Expert Interviews and Testimonials..105
Conclusion..**110**
References **114**

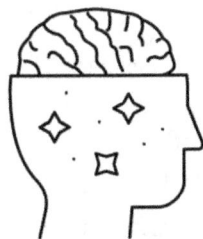

INTRODUCTION

Are you struggling to break free from addictive behaviors that have a hold on your life? In a world that's constantly buzzing with endless notifications, tempting distractions, and compelling habits, it's no wonder many of us find ourselves trapped in unhealthy routines that seem impossible to break. Whether you're someone who can't go more than a few minutes without checking your phone or you rely on late-night binge-watching sessions to unwind, the modern age has made it increasingly difficult to maintain a healthy balance of consuming content. That's where *The Dopamine Reset* comes into play as a practical guide designed to help you recalibrate your brain's reward system and achieve a balanced, fulfilling life.

Imagine waking up in the morning feeling refreshed, your mind clear and focused, without the overwhelming urge to scroll through social media or check your emails. You're able to engage in meaningful conversations with friends and family, fully present in the moment, without the distraction of your constantly buzzing phone. You finish your day with a sense of accomplishment and peace, rather than the guilt and frustration that often accompanies unproductive hours spent on addictive behaviors. This book aims to transform these visions into reality by offering you a comprehensive 21-day detox plan backed by proven insights and actionable strategies.

The unique approach of *The Dopamine Reset* lies in its focus on the brain's reward system—the complex network of neurons responsible for our experiences of pleasure and motivation. Many solutions for breaking free from addictive behaviors are merely temporary fixes. They might work for a short while, but they don't address the root cause of the problem. Our methodology delves deeper, providing you with tools to understand how and why your brain craves certain stimuli and offering sustainable ways to reset this system.

Over the next 21 days, you'll embark on a transformative journey filled with rewards and obstacles. You'll gradually eliminate overstimulating activities that hijack your brain's natural reward mechanisms and replace them with healthier habits that foster genuine well-being. Use this as an opportunity for a mental cleanse by giving yourself the chance to be rid of the mental clutter that's been holding you back from being the healthiest and most productive version of yourself.

Breaking free from deeply ingrained habits is never easy, and there will undoubtedly be moments when you feel tempted to revert to old patterns. Perhaps, you've previously tried to cut down your screen time or kick another unhealthy habit to the curb, only to find yourself back at square one after a few days. I understand how frustrating it can be to feel stuck in a cycle of addiction. That's why I wrote this book to offer you support, empathy, and practical advice to overcome each obstacle and trial of this journey.

This is a no-judgment zone, dedicated to helping you achieve long-term growth! You're not alone in this struggle. Whether you find yourself constantly glued to screens, battling unhealthy eating habits, or grappling with other addictive behaviors, *The Dopamine Reset—A 21-Day Detox* offers a clear path to reclaiming control and living a more mindful life.

Throughout these pages, you'll find a variety of exercises and techniques tailored to help you manage cravings, build resilience, and create lasting change. Each chapter is designed to guide you through specific aspects of the detox process, from understanding the science behind dopamine and addiction to implementing daily practices that promote mental well-being. By the end of the 21 days, you'll be able to break free from your most debilitating habits while using the valuable insights you've learned to maintain a balanced lifestyle.

You'll learn to replace mindless scrolling with mindful meditation, trade late-night snacking for nourishing meals, and swap out binge-watching for engaging in hobbies that bring you true joy and fulfillment. These changes won't just improve your mental health; they'll also enhance every aspect of your life, from your relationships and career to your overall sense of happiness and purpose.

This book isn't about perfection. Setbacks are a normal part of any transformative journey. What's important is how you respond to these challenges so that you can use them as opportunities for growth. With each passing day, you'll develop greater self-awareness and a stronger resolve, empowering you to make conscious choices that align with your goals and values.

Are you ready to take on the turbulent journey ahead of you that will be filled with challenging moments and rewarding experiences of change? By committing to this 21-day detox, you're making a powerful statement—to yourself and to the world—that you're ready to break free from the chains of addiction and embrace a healthier, happier lifestyle.

Get ready to change the way you think, feel, and live for the better! Together, we'll uncover the root causes of your addictive behaviors, equip you with the tools to overcome them, and celebrate every milestone along the way. The road to recovery starts here, and I couldn't be more excited to join you on this transformative adventure. Through these pages, you'll discover the remarkable potential that lies within you that you may not have been aware of.

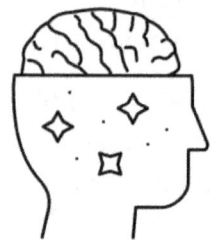

CHAPTER 1
Understanding Dopamine and Its Influence

You've heard all about dopamine and the powerful impact it has on us mentally and physically, but what is it exactly, and how is it able to influence us so strongly? Dopamine—a pivotal neurotransmitter in our brains—plays a crucial role in driving motivation, experiencing pleasure, and reinforcing behaviors. It serves as a chemical messenger that transmits signals between neurons, influencing everything from our moods to our decision-making processes. Grasping how dopamine functions can offer valuable insights into why we pursue certain activities and how various stimuli affect our brains.

In this chapter, we will delve into the intricate workings of dopamine, examining its definition, function, and significance in shaping our actions. We will explore how dopamine imbalances can impact mental health, highlighting links to conditions such as depression and Parkinson's disease. Additionally, we will discuss the connection between dopamine and addictive behaviors, shedding light on why some habits are challenging to break.

The Definition and Function of Dopamine

Let's determine what dopamine is and why it's crucial to understand when breaking free from addictive behaviors. Dopamine is one of the brain's most essential neurotransmitters, crucially involved in motivation, reward, and pleasure. Its functional role is to act as a messenger in your brain that releases signals between neurons. When released in various areas of the brain, it creates feelings of pleasure and satisfaction. These pleasurable sensations are the brain's way of encouraging us to repeat actions that are beneficial for survival, like eating and socializing.

Understanding the impact of dopamine on mood and behavior is fundamental to recognizing its broader influence on our daily lives. For instance, dopamine levels affect how we perceive rewards and can significantly sway our decision-making processes. Elevated dopamine levels generally lead to heightened feelings of happiness and satisfaction, while lower levels can result in apathy and lack of motivation. Dopamine imbalances have even been linked to conditions like depression and Parkinson's disease. In these scenarios, the deficiency of dopamine manifests in symptoms ranging from severe lack of motivation to significant motor control issues.

The Connection Between Dopamine and Addictive Behaviors

Dopamine releases feelings of reward when you consume substances. Whether this involves illicit drugs like heroin or everyday pleasures like eating sweet foods, dopamine communicates to your brain that these substances are rewarding you (Watson, 2021). The mesolimbic pathway—also known as the reward system—is heavily influenced here. When someone engages in a rewarding activity, this pathway is activated, leading to the release of dopamine and subsequent feelings of euphoria.

This same mechanism also explains why addictions form. Substances or activities that provide artificial surges of dopamine can hijack this reward system, causing individuals to associate the action with profound pleasure (Lewis et al., 2021). Over time, the repeated overstimulation causes tolerance, leading you to require higher doses to achieve the same effect and fostering dependence. Understanding this connection helps shed light on why breaking free from such addictions can be extraordinarily challenging.

How Dopamine Functions

A significant factor of dopamine is that the body makes and controls it naturally. The process starts with an amino acid called tyrosine, which the body turns into another substance called L-dopa, and then into dopamine through various chemical reactions. Eating foods high in tyrosine, like chicken, dairy, nuts, and soy, can help boost dopamine production, which might improve your mood and thinking skills.

Managing dopamine levels in the brain is quite complicated and involves several systems. A part of the brain called the striatum has many neurons that can either increase or decrease dopamine signals. It's crucial to keep these signals balanced to maintain the right amount of dopamine. If this balance is off, it can lead to problems like dopamine dysregulation syndrome, often seen in people being treated for Parkinson's disease.

Since dopamine plays a big role in mental health, learning how it works is essential for those wanting to feel better and break bad habits. There are many ways to keep dopamine levels in check such as regular exercise, good sleep, and other healthy activities. We will explore these strategies and some others in greater detail throughout the book.

How Dopamine Affects Motivation and Pleasure

Learning about the intricate relationship between dopamine, motivation, and pleasure reveals how this neurotransmitter plays a pivotal role in our behavior. Dopamine is often dubbed the "feel-good" chemical because it triggers the sensation of pleasure when we achieve or anticipate rewards. However, its functions extend far beyond just making us feel good; it is essential for influencing our motivation and goal-directed behavior.

Dopamine helps prepare your brain for action and gives you the push you need to pursue goals. This neurotransmitter acts as a catalyst that transforms your desires into tangible actions. When you set out to achieve something—whether it's finishing a project at work or sticking to a new exercise regimen—dopamine levels spike, which increases your focus and energy, propelling you toward your objective. Without adequate dopamine, you may struggle with initiating tasks or maintaining persistence, leading to challenges in productivity and accomplishing long-term goals.

One study by Lerner suggests that dopamine neurons are not a simple, uniform group; instead, they consist of various types that release dopamine under different circumstances, each with unique roles in motivation and behavior. The diverse roles of dopamine neurons showcase how this neurotransmitter has such an integral impact on our drive and behaviors (Northwestern Medicine, 2022). These findings emphasize that dopamine's role in motivation is not just about producing pleasure but also encouraging perseverance and effort in achieving goals.

Whenever we experience something pleasurable—like eating delicious food, receiving praise, or achieving a milestone—dopamine is released in the brain's reward system. This reinforces the behavior, making us more likely to repeat it. The brain associates the pleasurable feeling with the activity, creating a powerful feedback loop that encourages engagement in these rewarding behaviors. This mechanism is vital for learning and survival as it drives us to seek out beneficial experiences and avoid harmful ones.

However, the same processes that help reinforce positive behaviors can also lead to addiction. Addictive drugs exploit the dopamine system by causing massive dopamine releases, far beyond what natural rewards trigger. Over time, these surges can alter your brain's reward circuitry, making you crave your drug and find less joy in everyday activities. As highlighted in a study from Cell Reports led by Dr. Talia Lerner, compulsive reward-seeking behavior is promoted through heightened dopamine signaling, even when the outcomes are unpleasant (...Northwestern Medicine, 2022). This emphasizes the idea that addiction hijacks the brain's natural reward mechanisms, creating intense desire and compulsion that are hard to break.

Lerner's research also delves into how habits form and change within the dopamine system. Habits are initially goal-directed behaviors that become automated actions over time. For example, practicing a musical instrument starts as a deliberate activity driven by the desire to learn, but with repetition, it becomes a habit performed almost instinctively. Information we receive from various stimuli moves through the dopamine system into a part of our brain that is responsible for habit formation, the dorsolateral striatum. On the other hand, these habits can revert back to goal-directed behaviors if the brain circuits adapt accordingly. This two-way nature of dopamine circuits helps us understand how to break bad habits.

Given dopamine's powerful influence on our behavior, it's crucial to cultivate healthy sources of pleasure to avoid overstimulation. Chronic overstimulation—whether from addictive substances, excessive screen time, or indulgent foods—can desensitize the brain's reward system.

To maintain a balanced dopamine system, consider adopting strategies that encourage sustainable pleasure and motivation:

- **Engage in physical activity:** Regular exercise boosts dopamine production and enhances mood. Activities like running, swimming, and dancing provide natural rewards without the risk of overstimulation.

- **Pursue hobbies:** Engaging in creative activities such as painting, writing, or playing an instrument can stimulate dopamine release and foster long-term satisfaction.

- **Engage in healthy goal-directed behavior:** Follow SMART goals that are easy to set and follow. Each small achievement can trigger a dopamine release, keeping you motivated and focused.

- **Practice mindfulness and meditation:** Techniques such as mindfulness and meditation can help regulate dopamine levels, reducing stress and enhancing overall well-being.

- **Limit screen time**: Set boundaries for technology usage to prevent excessive dopamine spikes from social media and other digital distractions. Instead, spend time outdoors or with loved ones to foster genuine connections.

- **Ingest a healthy diet:** Consume foods rich in tyrosine, an amino acid that aids dopamine production. Foods like bananas, almonds, avocados, and lean meats can support healthy dopamine levels.

The Brain's Reward System Explained

Understanding how the brain processes rewards and the role of dopamine within this circuitry is crucial for grasping how our behaviors are shaped and habits are formed. At the center of this intricate system is the mesolimbic pathway, also known as the reward pathway. This pathway includes key brain regions such as the ventral tegmental area (VTA), the nucleus accumbens (NAcc), and parts of the prefrontal cortex. Each of these regions plays a vital role in how we perceive and respond to rewarding stimuli.

How the Brain's Reward System Works

The VTA is housed in the midbrain and serves as the starting point of the reward pathway. Neurons in the VTA release dopamine when they become activated by rewarding stimuli. These dopaminergic neurons project to the nucleus accumbens, which is part of the ventral striatum. The NAcc is often referred to as the brain's pleasure center because it's heavily involved in processing rewards and reinforcing pleasurable experiences. When dopamine is released into the NAcc, it creates feelings of euphoria and satisfaction.

From there, chemical messages are sent to the prefrontal cortex, where complex cognitive behavior—like decision-making and moderating social behavior—is controlled. This connection explains why rewards can significantly influence our choices and actions. For example, when you receive positive feedback at work, your prefrontal cortex helps you process this reward, leading to reinforced behavior such as increased productivity.

The Role of Dopamine in Reinforcing the Reward System

Dopamine isn't just responsible for making us seek out rewards but also makes sure we remember what to do to get those rewards again. This reinforcement mechanism is deeply rooted in our evolutionary biology. Natural rewards like food, water, and social interactions have historically been essential for survival, driving us to repeat behaviors that ensure we obtain these necessities.

However, there exists a downside to this powerful reinforcement system: Substances like alcohol, nicotine, and commonly abused drugs exploit this natural reward circuitry. They trigger massive surges of dopamine without providing any biological benefits, causing a strong reinforcement of drug-seeking behavior. According to neuropsychopharmacology expert Dr. Eliot L. Gardner (2011), addictive substances can hijack the brain's reward circuits, diverting a person's focus from natural pleasures to the pursuit of drug-induced euphoria.

But the story doesn't end with substances of abuse. Everyday activities can also lead to dopamine overstimulation if not kept in check. In our modern world, technology has become a major contributor to dopamine spikes. Each like or positive comment acts as a small reward, encouraging us to keep checking our devices.

To avoid falling into the trap of dopamine overstimulation, it is helpful to become aware of daily habits that contribute to this cycle. Throughout the further chapters, we will explore practical and effective ways to avoid dopamine overstimulation and addiction.

Key Takeaways of Dopamine and Its Influence

In this chapter, we have explored the intricate role of dopamine in our behavior, highlighting its influence on motivation, pleasure, and decision-making. By acknowledging how dopamine levels affect our mood and actions, we gain insight into the neurological underpinnings of both healthy behaviors and addictive tendencies. Knowledge of the brain's reward system, including key regions like the VTA and NAcc, helps us see why certain activities and substances can create powerful habits and dependencies.

Recognizing how dopamine functions allows us to make informed choices that support our mental well-being, leading to a more balanced and fulfilling life not run by dopamine. We are unable to make changes in our lifestyle to balance our dopamine if we aren't aware of the issue at hand. Being able to recognize addictive behavior is the first step toward resetting your dopamine clock. In the next chapter, we will uncover all the signs and symptoms of addiction that you may be unaware of.

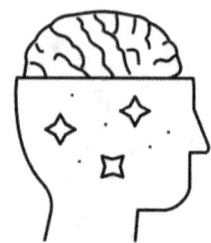

CHAPTER 2
Recognizing Your Addictive Behaviors

You've been noticing a change in your mood, ability to focus, and overall well-being, but you're not sure what's causing such an overwhelmingly negative strain on your life. We can often only identify our toxic and addictive behaviors once they've already gotten a grip on us. Many individuals unknowingly engage in habits that trigger the brain's reward system, setting them on a path toward addiction. This chapter explores how certain behaviors can lead to an unhealthy dependence on dopamine. Understanding how these behaviors manifest is the first step in identifying and addressing potential addictions.

This chapter delves into various facets of addictive behaviors, breaking down their psychological and emotional impacts. It examines how excessive dopamine can disrupt decision-making processes, emotional stability, and cognitive functions like memory and concentration. In addition to these mental and emotional effects, the physical symptoms of dopamine imbalance, including restlessness and insomnia, showcase the multifaceted nature of addiction. By recognizing these signs, you can develop effective strategies to manage and overcome your addictive behaviors.

Symptoms of Dopamine Dependence

Learning about the signs of dopamine dependence and its impact on behavior is essential for breaking free from unhealthy habits. When dopamine is released, the behaviors you're participating in at that moment are reinforced, making you compelled to repeat them. As we've established, it doesn't only form beneficial routines; it can also lead to addiction when dopamine levels become dysregulated. These are common symptoms and signs that you're experiencing dopamine dependence or dysregulation:

- **Behavioral signs:** Behavioral impacts are one of the first indicators to look for when recognizing dopamine dependence. Excessive dopamine can significantly affect decision-making and impulsivity. For instance, you might find yourself making rash decisions, opting for immediate gratification over healthier long-term benefits. This can manifest in various ways, such as compulsive shopping, overeating, or excessive use of technology. These behaviors are often promoted by the brain's reinforcement of the activity, making it harder to resist despite knowing the negative consequences. Many people with high dopamine activity also struggle with self-control, making it difficult for them to stick to plans or goals, which can lead to a vicious cycle of poor decision-making that perpetuates the addictive behavior.

- **Emotional symptoms:** Emotional patterns provide another window into our knowledge of dopamine dependence. Having a dopamine imbalance can contribute to mood swings and emotional instability. High dopamine levels are often associated with feelings of euphoria and heightened energy, but this can quickly turn into anxiety, stress, or irritability when dopamine levels drop. These fluctuations can create an emotional roller coaster, driving you to seek out activities or substances that boost your dopamine levels to regain a sense of well-being. For example, after the initial high from drug use wears off, the individual might feel anxious or depressed, prompting them to use again to alleviate these unpleasant emotions (NIDA, 2020). This cycle not only exacerbates emotional instability but also reinforces the dependency on the addictive substance or behavior, causing a never-ending loop.

- **Cognitive impact:** The cognitive effects of dopamine dysregulation can also be a telling sign of dopamine addiction. Dopamine plays an important role in our cognitive abilities such as attention span and memory. An imbalance of dopamine can have a negative influence on these basic cognitive functions. You may find it hard to concentrate, experience "brain fog," or have trouble remembering things. This cognitive impairment can be particularly challenging for tasks that require sustained mental effort or critical thinking. Over time, the brain can become less sensitive to natural rewards, making it harder to find pleasure in everyday activities. This diminished sensitivity can lead to a lack of motivation and a feeling of lifelessness, pushing you to further seek high-dopamine activities to feel normal (Dellwo, 2023).

- **Physical signs:** Physical manifestations are also common signs of dopamine dysregulation. Symptoms like restlessness, insomnia, or even physical discomfort can be caused by issues with dopamine levels. Restlessness and a constant need for stimulation often accompany high dopamine activity, making it difficult for you to relax or sit still. Insomnia occurs because elevated dopamine levels can interfere with the body's natural sleep-wake cycle. This lack of sleep not only affects physical health but also contributes to emotional and cognitive difficulties. Physical discomfort or pain can also arise, as the brain's altered reward system no longer signals pleasure from typical activities, leading to a pervasive sense of unease.

Because dopamine is so deeply embedded in our brain's reward system, its dysregulation can ripple through every aspect of our lives, affecting how we think, feel, and act. Identifying these signs early and understanding their impact is the first step toward breaking free from addictive behaviors.

Assessing Technology Addiction

Let's start by evaluating technology dependency and the influence it has on our dopamine levels. Digital addiction is extremely prevalent in our current age, when social media, television, and all forms of technology have evolved to become hard to resist.

Screen Time Analysis

Technology has become integrated into each aspect of our lives, which can be both positive and negative. From smartphones to computers, we are constantly connected, often without realizing the extent of our screen usage. Assessing your screen time is crucial for understanding its impact on dopamine release in your brain. When we use technology—particularly social media and video games—our brains release dopamine, creating a sense of euphoria similar to what one might experience with certain addictive substances.

To begin addressing technology dependency, you should start by monitoring your daily screen time. Most of our devices have a feature where we can view our usage patterns. For instance, smartphones offer weekly updates summarizing how much time you've spent on various apps. Keeping tabs on these metrics can help you identify any excessive or potentially harmful usage.

Behavioral Patterns

Identifying compulsive behaviors related to technology is another key aspect of recognizing technology addiction. Compulsive behavior manifests through an irresistible urge to engage with screens, even when it interferes with other important aspects of life. Signs of addiction include prioritizing screen time over face-to-face interactions, family activities, or hobbies once enjoyed. For example, your children or younger siblings might choose screens over playing outside, reading books, or engaging in creative play.

If you find yourself compulsively checking your phone, scrolling through social media late into the night, or experiencing anxiety when separated from your device, these could be red flags indicating a deeper issue. Another behavioral indicator is the inability to reduce screen time despite repeated attempts. If the struggle to cut back leads to feelings of irritability or restlessness, it might suggest a dependency. At this point, setting clear boundaries around technology use is imperative.

Impact on Well-Being

Technology addiction can have significant repercussions on mental well-being. Prolonged exposure to digital devices can lead to increased stress, anxiety, and even depression. Constant notifications and the urge to stay updated can overwhelm the brain, leading to mental fatigue and burnout (Nakshine et al., 2022).

Being on social media frequently can cause feelings of loneliness and inadequacy due to comparing ourselves to other people's seemingly perfect social, professional, and personal lives. This can further contribute to poor mental health, as you become more likely to develop low self-esteem and negative thought patterns. Children and teenagers are particularly susceptible to these effects, as their developing brains and social skills are heavily influenced by their online experiences.

To avoid the negative impacts of social media, it's important to develop a healthy relationship with the digital world. If this is a household issue and your children are also impacted, encourage open conversations about the content consumed online, emphasizing critical thinking and mindfulness. Promote activities that enhance real-world connections and emotional well-being, such as engaging in hobbies and spending quality time with each other.

Detox Necessity

Recognizing the need for a digital detox is vital for maintaining overall health and balance. A digital detox involves taking a deliberate break from screens to reset your brain's reward system and reduce dependency on technology. The goal is to restore a sense of equilibrium where technology is used intentionally rather than impulsively.

It's important to have realistic goals and expectations for your detox so that you aren't too hard on yourself throughout this turbulent journey. Begin small and gradually increase your goals. You can implement screen-free periods during specific times of the day, such as the first hour after waking up or the last hour before bed. Appreciate your time offline by engaging in activities that are fulfilling to you.

Encouraging friends and family to join you in a digital detox can create a supportive environment. Share your experiences and strategies for managing cravings and staying committed to reducing screen time. Overcoming technology addiction requires patience and persistence, but the benefits of improved mental well-being and a healthier lifestyle make it a worthwhile endeavor.

Unhealthy Eating Patterns

Identifying detrimental eating habits that can contribute to dopamine dysregulation is crucial for anyone looking to improve their overall mental and physical health. When our eating habits interfere with dopamine regulation, it can lead to addictive behaviors similar to those seen with substance abuse. Factors that negatively contribute to unhealthy eating behaviors include the following:

- **Intense food cravings:** Food cravings are one of the primary indicators of how certain foods can influence dopamine release in the brain. Energy-dense foods—particularly those rich in sugars and fats—are known to trigger dopamine production, making them highly appealing. The repeated consumption of these delicious and tempting foods reinforces their pleasurable effects, creating a cycle of craving and indulgence. Studies have shown that such foods can significantly alter dopamine pathways, contributing to overeating and obesity (Fuente González et al., 2022). To break this cycle, it's essential to identify and manage food cravings. One way to do this is by keeping a food diary to track what you eat and how you feel afterward, helping you recognize patterns and triggers.

- **Emotional eating:** Emotional eating is another detrimental habit that many people fall into without realizing its impact on dopamine levels. You may find yourself turning to food to cope with stress, sadness, or other negative emotions. This form of eating provides temporary relief but can lead to long-term issues such as weight gain and more profound emotional distress. Research indicates a strong relationship between negative emotional states and the consumption of unhealthy, high-calorie foods (Bennett et al., 2013). Identifying the difference between physical hunger cues and emotional hunger responses can help you manage your emotional eating. Techniques that promote mindfulness, such as journaling and meditation, can help you address the underlying emotional triggers without resorting to food.

- **Unhealthy dietary choices:** The nutritional impact of your diet also plays a significant role in dopamine regulation. Poor dietary choices—particularly those lacking in essential nutrients—can impair the functioning of dopamine receptors and disrupt neurotransmitter balance. Regularly consuming foods high in sugar can negatively impact your mood by causing drastic spikes and subsequent crashes in your blood sugar levels. A well-balanced diet ensures that your body receives the necessary nutrients to produce and regulate neurotransmitters effectively, promoting holistic well-being. We will explore nutritious well-balanced meal alternatives further into our detox journey.

- **Negatively influential mealtime routines:** Mealtime rituals and routines can also contribute to unhealthy eating behaviors related to dopamine dysregulation. Regularly eating meals at inconsistent times, skipping meals, or eating in front of screens can all disrupt natural hunger and satiety cues. Establishing a consistent mealtime routine helps regulate your body's internal clock, reducing the likelihood of overeating or indulging in unhealthy snacks. Taking the time to savor your food without distractions can also improve digestion and make mealtime a more enjoyable and mindful experience. Try setting specific times for breakfast, lunch, and dinner, and avoid multitasking while eating to fully engage with your food.

If you notice these signs of unhealthy eating patterns, a dopamine detox can transform your relationship with food, by helping you savor and appreciate the nutrients your body needs to thrive, instead of using food as a means to feed your emotions.

Substance Abuse and Other Addictive Behaviors

Recognizing the warning signs of substance abuse and other addictive behaviors is an essential step in breaking free from harmful patterns that are detrimental to your safety and quality of life. To begin with, it is important to identify substances known to influence dopamine levels, as these can lead to addiction. Common substances include inhalants, opioids (including prescription and nonprescription), stimulants like Adderall and methamphetamine, and nicotine products like cigarettes or e-cigarettes. These substances strongly activate the brain's reward center, producing feelings of pleasure that can drive repetitive use and, ultimately, addiction. Alcohol addiction is a prevalent issue globally amongst various age groups, affecting about 10% of people aged 12 or older in the US (Cleveland Clinic, 2023).

Signs of addictive behavior are just as concerning. This includes activities that stimulate your brain's reward system, turning this pleasurable behavior into a habit that's hard to let go of. Some activities that can have this stimulating effect include overeating, gambling, exercising, shopping, video gaming, having sex, and using the internet. Behavioral scientists have noted similarities between substance and behavioral addictions, particularly how both disrupt daily functioning. Gambling disorder, for example, is currently recognized in the DSM-5 as a diagnosable behavioral addiction due to extensive research on its impacts (Cleveland Clinic, 2023). It's important to note that activities that aren't officially identified and recognized as addiction disorders are still valid, as any addictive behavior will have a significant mental, social, and physical impact on your welfare.

Ways to Navigate Addiction

A crucial step in managing addiction is risk assessment, which involves evaluating personal behaviors for potential addictive tendencies. This process begins with self-reflection and monitoring your habits. Follow these tips to navigate your addiction the best way you can:

- **Identify warning signs:** Warning signs of addiction often include an inability to stop using a substance or engaging in an activity despite the desire to do so. People may find themselves lying to loved ones about their usage or attempting to hide it. Increased tolerance is another red flag; over time, more of the substance or activity is needed to achieve the same euphoric effects. An intense focus on the addiction, where it takes over one's life and thoughts, also points to a problem. Individuals might feel they've lost complete control, often experiencing guilt, depression, or helplessness due to addiction-related impacts. Experiencing withdrawal symptoms after reducing the use of an addictive substance or behavior is a telltale sign of being addicted and out of control (*Signs and Symptoms of Addiction*, n.d.).

- **Evaluate personal risk:** When evaluating personal risks, consider whether your routines revolve excessively around certain substances or activities. Keeping a journal to track frequency and intensity can help highlight problematic patterns. Reflect on moments when you've chosen an addictive behavior over important responsibilities or relationships. Assess how often you think about or crave the substance or activity during your daily life. Honest self-assessment is vital for recognizing the potential for addiction before it becomes severe.

- **Seek professional help:** Finally, seeking help is an essential aspect of addressing addictive behaviors. Recognizing when professional intervention or support is necessary can make a significant difference in recovery. If you find yourself unable to stop using a substance or engaging in an activity despite multiple attempts, don't hesitate to seek help. The journey to recovery often requires external support, whether from healthcare professionals, support groups, or close friends and family. Support systems provide accountability, coping strategies, and encouragement, which are all crucial for overcoming addiction.

When considering professional intervention, look for resources such as addiction counselors, therapists, or rehabilitation programs. Many communities offer support groups like Alcoholics Anonymous (AA) or Narcotics Anonymous (NA), which create a network of individuals who share similar experiences. Becoming a part of these groups helps you find a sense of belonging that makes you feel understood. This can make the recovery process less daunting and isolating. Additionally, healthcare providers can offer medical treatments or therapies designed to manage withdrawal symptoms and reduce cravings.

Do You Recognize Your Addictive Behaviors?

We have delved into the complex world of dopamine dependence, identifying various habits that can lead to addiction. By examining behavioral impacts, emotional patterns, cognitive effects, and physical manifestations, we have painted a comprehensive picture of how excessive dopamine influences our lives. Recognizing these signs early can pave the way for developing effective strategies to manage dopamine levels and break free from addictive behaviors.

Awareness of the underlying science behind your brain's reward system and dopamine empowers you to seek healthier alternatives that provide similar rewards without harmful consequences. Seeking help and guidance from professionals is a vital part of the recovery process. With these insights, you have gained the mindfulness needed to identify addictive behaviors in your lifestyle. What addiction gives you a dopamine rush that you depend on, and why do you think you need to detox from it to improve your happiness and quality of life? In the next chapter, we will dive into the preparations you'll need to practice before starting your 21-day detox.

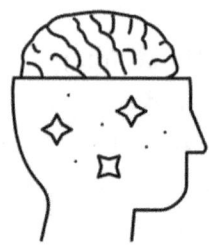

CHAPTER 3
Preparing for Your 21-Day Detox

You've identified your unhealthy attachment to dopamine, and you want to change your quality of life for the better. You're ready for a reset, so you can start appreciating the small pleasures in life. But before you start your 21-day detox, it's important to set up a fitting environment for success. The space where you spend most of your time can significantly impact your mental state and overall progress during the detox period. By making mindful adjustments to your living conditions, you can create a foundation that supports positive habits and helps you maintain focus throughout this transformative journey.

This chapter will guide you through creating a supportive environment tailored to your detox needs. Additionally, we'll explore mindful consumption practices that involve being deliberate about the media, information, and food you consume. Each of these elements plays a fundamental role in setting the stage for an effective and fulfilling dopamine detox experience.

Creating a Supportive Environment

Creating a successful detox experience begins with establishing surroundings that promote positive habits.

Organizing Your Space

To achieve mental clarity and focus, it's vital to be surrounded by a clutter-free environment. Clutter can be overwhelming and distracting, making it difficult to concentrate on the goals of your detox. Start by decluttering the areas where you spend the most time, such as your bedroom, kitchen, and living room. Sort through your belongings, remove unnecessary items, and opt for a minimalist approach where possible. Keep only what you need and cherish, and donate and let go of what you no longer need. This helps to create a calm and ordered atmosphere.

It's also incredibly helpful to reorganize your workspace to foster productivity. Ensure that your desk is tidy and free of distractions by using storage solutions like drawers, shelves, and organizers to keep essentials within reach while avoiding clutter. Adding elements that inspire you—such as motivational quotes or personal mementos—can enhance the ambiance and boost your motivation throughout the detox.

Creating a Schedule

Developing a structured routine that aligns with your detox goals can provide consistency and support new habits. Begin by outlining your daily activities and prioritizing tasks that contribute to your detox objectives. Add a fixed timeline that includes when you eat your meals, exercise, work, relax, and sleep. Having a clear structure reduces decision fatigue and helps maintain discipline. The following tips can help you set a daily schedule that works for you:

- Plan your mornings mindfully. Starting the day with meditation, breathing exercises, or light physical activity can set a positive tone for the rest of the day.

- Consider incorporating practices like gratitude journaling, where you write down three things you're grateful for each morning. Journaling shifts your focus away from negative self-talk that influences a loop of addictive behavior and instead encourages mental and emotional well-being.

- Plan sufficient breaks in your schedule, and use these moments to rest and recharge. Ensure that you have a chance to step away from screens and engage in activities that bring joy and relaxation, such as walking in nature, listening to music, or connecting with loved ones.

Consistently following a structured routine helps reinforce healthy habits and creates a smoother transition into a detoxified lifestyle.

Practicing Mindful Consumption

Mindful consumption involves being deliberate about the information you absorb and the food choices you make. In the modern fast-paced world, where we are constantly bombarded with stimuli, we can often find ourselves feeling mentally exhausted and stressed. It's important to filter out unnecessary noise and focus on consuming content that enriches your life.

When it comes to information and media, choose quality over quantity. Limit exposure to negative news by selecting credible sources and allocating specific times for catching up on current events. Choose to consume content that motivates and educates you. Engage with information that inspires, educates, and uplifts you. For instance, listen to podcasts that teach new skills or watch documentaries that broaden your horizons.

Mindful food consumption is just as important. Opt for nutritious, whole foods that support your body's natural detox processes. Plan and prepare balanced meals that make you feel nourished and energized. Avoid processed foods and excessive sugar, as they can trigger a dopamine imbalance that hinders your detox efforts. Practicing mindful eating exercises, such as the one below, can help you make better food choices while finding joy and appreciation in simple and balanced meals:

1. Take your food to a calm environment, and sit down at a table.
2. Practice some deep breathing before starting your meal to bring your full attention to your current moment.
3. Appreciate your food by acknowledging all the effort that was put into it.
4. Start eating your food, and purposefully observe and enjoy the flavors, smells, and textures of each bite.
5. Listen to your body when it's sending cues that you're full.

By being mindful of what you consume, you create a balanced environment conducive to your detox goals. This practice extends beyond food to encompass all aspects of life, promoting greater awareness and intentionality in everyday choices. In later chapters, we'll discuss some alternative daily practices and routines that could also benefit from mindfulness techniques!

Detox Essentials and Supplies

To have a successful dopamine detox journey, prepare yourself with the essentials and supplies that can help you stay accountable and disciplined as you avoid addictive behavior. The following are some valuable essentials to keep handy before your detox reset:

- **Journaling materials:** An essential tool for optimizing your detox experience is reflective journaling. Keeping a journal allows you to document your progress, emotions, and insights throughout the detox period. This practice not only helps in tracking changes and improvements but also provides an outlet for self-reflection and emotional release. Consider using notebooks that appeal to you visually, as an inviting journal can make the act of writing more enjoyable. You might also explore structured journaling prompts focused on wellness and personal growth to guide your reflections. As you journal, note any patterns or triggers related to dopamine dependency, and record how your feelings evolve during the detox process. This valuable continuous feedback can support lasting behavioral change.

- **Healthy snacks and meals:** Nourishing your body with nutritional meals can improve your energy levels while on a detox. Stocking up on healthy snacks and meals can help maintain your physical health and boost mental clarity. Prioritize whole foods like fresh fruits and vegetables, nuts, seeds, and lean proteins. Preparing meal plans in advance can prevent the temptation of reaching for unhealthy options when you're hungry. Consider incorporating recipes that are both nutritious and easy to prepare, ensuring you spend minimal time in the kitchen. Staying hydrated is equally important; aim to drink plenty of water throughout the day to keep your body functioning optimally.

- **Relaxation aids:** Incorporating relaxation aids can significantly enhance your detox journey, providing moments of calm and helping to manage stress. Create a calm atmosphere by using tools like candles, essential oils, and tranquil music. Essential oils like lavender, chamomile, or eucalyptus can be used as a form of aromatherapy that promotes a relaxing environment that helps you achieve better quality sleep. Mindfulness exercises—including deep breathing, meditation, and light stretching—can also be beneficial. Establishing a bedtime routine that includes these relaxation aids can improve your sleep hygiene, further supporting your detox efforts.

By equipping yourself with these tools and resources, you lay a solid foundation for a transformative detox experience. The strategic use of relaxation tools helps break the cycle of dopamine dependence, while reflective journaling fosters deeper self-awareness and accountability.

Engaging in a dopamine detox requires commitment and intentional actions. When you choose to use your devices during this dopamine reset, ensure you put proper measures in place to avoid the temptation to doomscroll. Configure your devices so they encourage productive habits rather than hinder them.

Setting Realistic Goals and Expectations

Setting the stage for a successful detox involves establishing achievable targets and understanding the detox process for long-term success. One effective method to accomplish this is through SMART goal setting. Using this structured approach provides clarity and direction, making it easier to stay focused and motivated. Here is how you can go about using SMART goals to enhance the results of your dopamine reset:

- **Specific goals** are clear and precise, outlining exactly what you aim to achieve during your detox. For example, rather than stating, "I want to reduce my screen time," a specific goal would be, "I will limit my screen time to two hours per day." This specificity helps to remove any ambiguity, providing a clear target to work toward.

- **Measurable goals** build awareness of your progress and how close you are to completing a goal. By keeping track of your accomplishments, you can celebrate small victories that motivate you to continue. For instance, if your goal is to meditate daily for 10 minutes daily, use a journal or an app to record each session. This tangible evidence of progress can bolster your confidence and commitment to the dopamine detox process (*Achieving Sobriety with SMART Goals...*, 2024).

- **Achievable goals** are realistic and within reach, taking into account your current capabilities and resources. It's important not to set yourself up for failure by aiming too high. Start with smaller goals to help you achieve those larger and more daunting goals. For example, if you want to incorporate exercise into your routine but haven't been active recently, start with a goal of walking for 15 minutes each day, gradually increasing the duration as you build your stamina.

- **Relevant goals** align with your values, needs, and aspirations, ensuring they are meaningful and impactful. They should reflect your personal motivations for undergoing the dopamine detox. Question the importance of each goal for achieving your holistic fulfillment and dreams. For example, limiting screen time might be relevant if you're looking to reduce stress and improve sleep quality.

- **Time-bound goals** utilize timeframes to promote a sense of urgency and accountability. Setting deadlines prompts action and helps prioritize efforts. For instance, instead of aiming to reduce screen time indefinitely, set a goal to achieve your desired limit within one month. This way, you have a clear endpoint to measure your progress.

Managing your expectations is just as important as setting transformative goals. It's important to be realistic to avoid disappointment and promote patience and self-compassion. Consider the following when setting expectations for your dopamine reset:

- **Realize there will be challenges:** Understanding the potential challenges and withdrawal symptoms you may face during your detox is crucial for mental preparedness. Detoxing from technology or other high-dopamine habits can lead to discomfort as your body and mind adjust. Some symptoms people often experience include restlessness, irritability, and difficulty concentrating. Recognizing these challenges ahead of time allows you to develop strategies to cope with them effectively.

- **Find strategies to manage withdrawals:** To help you navigate the obstacle of withdrawal, plan ahead with effective techniques to reduce stressful symptoms. One way to do this is to prepare alternative activities that can keep you engaged and distracted. Engage in your favorite hobbies to fill the void left by reduced dopamine-surging activities. Also, consider reaching out to friends and family for support when you feel the urge to revert to old habits. Surrounding yourself with a supportive network can offer encouragement and accountability.

- **Track your goals:** Implementing progress-tracking methods is another key aspect of a successful detox journey. Keeping a journal can help you monitor your behavior providing you with valuable insights into your patterns, which allows you to identify areas to improve. Regularly monitoring your progress allows you to make necessary adjustments so that you stay on track and continue making progress. For example, if your goal is to meditate daily, maintain a log of each meditation session. Note the duration, your feelings before and after meditating, and any challenges you encountered. This practice can help you observe trends and make informed decisions about how to enhance your routine.

- **Be patient:** Cultivating patience and resilience is essential as change takes time, and setbacks may occur. Understand that progress is not always linear, and there may be days when you struggle to adhere to your goals. Rather than becoming discouraged, view setbacks as learning opportunities. Reflect on what triggered the lapse and how you can address similar situations in the future. Find suitable personalized practices that help you stay grounded and focused, reducing the likelihood of impulsive reactions.

It's beneficial to set realistic expectations and remind yourself that significant change often comes gradually. Comparing your progress to others can undermine your efforts, so focus on your individual journey. Celebrate your unique achievements, and recognize the effort invested in your detox process.

Involving Friends and Family for Support

Engaging social connections to enhance accountability and encouragement during the detox is a cornerstone for success. Detoxing—whether from technology, unhealthy habits, or substances—is a massive lifestyle shift. This journey can often feel isolating, so developing a healthy support network can make this experience feel less daunting and lonely.

Building a Support Network

Creating a multifaceted support network begins with communicating your detox goals to your loved ones. By sharing your intentions, you invite them to understand and support your journey. Doing this can build trust and companionship with people in your support system, while providing you with additional support throughout your detox journey(*How to Rebuild Your Life: Strategies for Long-Term Recovery*, 2024).

Start by identifying key individuals in your life who will be supportive. These might include family members, close friends, or colleagues who understand the importance of your detox. Open communication about your goals and progress fosters transparency and invites genuine encouragement. For example, if you're aiming to reduce your screen time, inform your family about this goal so they can help you avoid distractions and offer positive reinforcement when you stick to your plan.

When discussing your detox goals with loved ones, be clear and specific about what you hope to achieve. Have conversations about your detox so that they can understand why it's so important to you. You can also explain the ways in which you'll need their support throughout the detox. Your honesty will encourage them to be more understanding and involved, making it easier for you to stay committed.

Accountability Partners

An accountability partner can reinforce your detox needs in moments when you want to give up. This person can be a friend or a family member who either participates in the detox with you or regularly checks in to provide encouragement and support. Partnering with someone who understands your challenges can make the journey less daunting and more enjoyable.

For example, if both you and a close friend decide to limit your social media usage, you can motivate each other and share progress. Regular check-ins can affirm your commitment to the detox and keep you both accountable. You might set up weekly meetings to discuss your experiences, struggles, and triumphs, creating a sense of shared purpose.

Choose an accountability partner who is reliable, trustworthy, and genuinely interested in your well-being. Establish a routine for check-ins that works for both of you, whether it's daily text messages or weekly coffee meet-ups. The consistency of this routine will boost your resolve and provide ongoing motivation.

Seeking Professional Help

Seeking professional help is also vital for those struggling with severe dopamine dysregulation. Therapies like cognitive behavioral therapy—which we will discuss in Chapter 7—can help reframe thought patterns and change behaviors that contribute to addiction. Medical treatments may also be necessary in cases where dopamine dysregulation has led to significant mental health issues or physical symptoms. In such instances, a healthcare provider can offer medications that help balance dopamine levels and improve overall quality of life.

Be aware of the severity of your addiction issues so you're able to identify when you need professional intervention. A professional psychologist or therapist can also be a valuable tool to make use of throughout your detox journey, regardless of how severe your addiction is.

Communication Strategies

Effective communication with those around you is vital as you embark on your detox. Setting clear boundaries and expectations with your close relationships can foster a supportive environment. Discussing these boundaries ensures that everyone understands and respects the changes you're implementing, reducing potential conflicts or misunderstandings.

For instance, if your detox involves cutting back on work-related emails after hours, communicate this boundary to your colleagues and supervisors. Explain the reasons behind this decision, and outline how you'll manage work responsibilities within set hours. Similarly, if you need quiet time for activities like meditation or reading, let your household know so they can respect this personal space.

Use assertive yet respectful language when setting boundaries. Be open and honest without seeming rude or confrontational. For example, you might say, "I've decided to limit my screen time in the evenings to improve my mental well-being. I hope you can support me by not expecting immediate responses to messages after 7 p.m."

Celebrating Progress

Don't forget to share special moments of progress with your support system so that they can celebrate milestones with you. These celebrations can take many forms, from simple acknowledgments and words of encouragement to more tangible rewards like a special outing or a treat.

For instance, if you've successfully avoided unnecessary screen time for a week, share this accomplishment with your partner or family. Their congratulations can bolster your confidence and remind you that your efforts are noticed and valued. Similarly, acknowledging your successes at support group meetings can be a way of accessing additional encouragement and inspiration.

Sharing your progress can also involve documenting your journey through journaling or social media updates (if relevant to your goals), allowing others to witness your growth. This transparency can even inspire members of your support network to embark on their own journeys toward healthier habits.

How to Prepare for Your Dopamine Reset

In this chapter, we explored the importance of creating a supportive environment for a successful detox. We discussed organizing your living space to promote clarity and focus, setting boundaries with technology to minimize distractions, creating a structured daily schedule to foster new habits, and practicing mindful consumption of both media and food. These strategies are designed to help you maintain a balanced life while minimizing stress and boosting your overall well-being during your dopamine detox journey.

As you move forward, remember that progress is key. Celebrate your commitment to this detox with all the important people in your life. With all of these practices at hand, you're ready to embrace a healthier and more fulfilling lifestyle. Starting your 21-day detox will help you unlearn your unhealthy habits and build new, long-lasting ones. In the next chapter, we will begin the 21-day detox, and I'll walk you through the first week of your transformative journey.

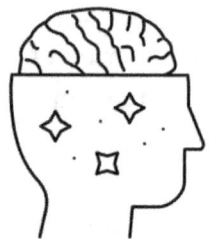

CHAPTER 4
Week 1—Eliminating Overstimulating Activities

You're now mentally, physically, and emotionally prepared for the transformative journey that lies ahead. Let's dive into week one and all the strategies and exercises you should follow to have a successful start to your detox. Eliminating overstimulating activities is one such crucial practice for enhancing mental well-being and achieving a more balanced lifestyle.

In this chapter, we will explore effective strategies to cut out activities that cause these dopamine spikes. Various practical steps are outlined to help you reduce technological dependence in your daily life. You'll also discover some fun alternative activities that can replace the time you used to spend on your screens, which can help you develop a healthier daily routine.

Techniques for Unplugging From Technology

When your mind and body have grown so attached to consuming multiple types of media and online content a day, it can make you feel purposeless to go without your technology. It's essential to take deliberate steps to manage your screen time and mitigate the overstimulation caused by constant digital engagement. This section offers practical strategies to reduce technology-driven dopamine spikes and crashes.

Implementing Digital Detox Practices

One of the most effective ways to begin reducing technology overstimulation is by implementing digital detox practices. A digital detox involves intentionally reducing or eliminating the use of digital devices for a set period, which can bring numerous benefits such as improved mental clarity, reduced stress, and better sleep quality.

It's important to start with a concise vision for your detox experience. Identify why you want to reduce your tech use and what positive changes you hope to achieve. Establish whether you want to partially reduce digital use or eliminate it from your daily life altogether. Then, set specific targets, such as reducing your daily screen time by two hours or avoiding screens entirely after 8 p.m. Research suggests that even brief periods away from digital devices can significantly alleviate stress and enhance overall well-being (*Digital Detox*, 2024).

Additionally, try to limit unnecessary background screen usage, such as having the TV on while doing other activities. By consciously reducing passive screen time, you can create a healthier relationship with technology. If you do choose to watch TV or use your phone in moderation, make sure you're doing so mindfully and intentionally.

Plan your digital detox carefully. Prepare mentally for the change by informing family and friends about your intentions so that they know why you might not respond to messages promptly. You can start by reducing your hourly screen time each day. Gradually increase the length of your digital detox periods to make the transition smoother and more sustainable in the long term. Reflect on your digital detox experiences, and make any adjustments needed to incorporate these new habits into daily life.

Creating Technology-Free Zones

Designating specific areas in your home as technology-free zones can also help reduce overstimulation. These spaces should be dedicated to relaxation and mindfulness, free from the distractions of digital devices.

Banning tech devices in your bedroom can significantly improve your sleep quality because the blue light emitted from screens can interfere with your production of melatonin—the hormone that regulates your sleep. By removing devices from the bedroom, you create an environment conducive to restful sleep.

Similarly, you could designate the dining area as a place for meals and conversation without the interruption of phones or tablets. This practice encourages more mindful eating and fosters stronger connections with family members. Doing this can help you have more meaningful interactions with your family, instead of being consumed by your devices.

Setting Specific Time Limits for Social Media and Device Usage

To control the amount of time spent on devices, set specific limits for social media and other forms of digital engagement. Establish boundaries for when and how long you will use these platforms. For example, you can restrict social media activity to 30 minutes per day or only during certain times, such as during lunch breaks or after dinner.

In this digital age, apps, timers, and software can facilitate screen time management and help in reducing digital distractions. Applications like Forest and StayFocusd allow users to block distracting websites for set periods, fostering productivity and encouraging breaks from screens. Using built-in features on smartphones, such as the "Screen Time" feature on iOS or "Digital Wellbeing" on Android, can provide insights into daily usage and help set limits. Timers and reminders can also prompt you to take regular breaks and engage in non-digital activities, aiding in maintaining a balanced routine.

Make use of the different features your phone has. You can block notification banners from specific apps, as they may be a tempting distraction. Don't be afraid to switch off your phone and place it out of sight and mind during specific times of the day. Doing this at night can be a valuable routine. This practice allows the mind to unwind before bedtime, leading to better sleep quality and reduced stress levels.

Healthy Food Alternatives

Healthier eating habits play a crucial role in regulating dopamine levels, which is essential for maintaining optimal mental well-being. By making conscious choices about the foods we consume, we can support our brain health and avoid items that cause overstimulation and lead to dopamine spikes. Let's uncover several ways to cultivate better nutrition practices to aid you along your first week of change:

- **Adapt to a more balanced diet:** Our dietary habits significantly impact how our brains function, influencing mood, cognitive abilities, and resistance to stress. Opting for whole foods and nutrient-dense meals ensures that the brain gets the necessary nutrients to operate efficiently. Whole foods, such as vegetables, fruits, and whole grains, can provide you with all the nutrients and antioxidants your body requires to function optimally. Dark green leafy vegetables like spinach and kale are particularly beneficial due to their high content of brain-protective compounds (Sutter Health, 2019). Similarly, omega-3 fatty acids, found in fish, have been shown to enhance brain health by reducing inflammation and promoting neuron growth. Incorporating lean proteins, complex carbohydrates, and healthy fats into your daily diet forms the backbone of well-balanced meals. Lean proteins, including poultry, fish, beans, and eggs, supply amino acids like tyrosine and tryptophan, which are precursors for neurotransmitters such as dopamine and serotonin, helping to regulate mood, sleep, and appetite (Walker, 2024). Complex carbohydrates—found in whole grains, sweet potatoes, and legumes—provide a slow and steady release of glucose to the brain, supporting sustained mental energy instead of the sharp spikes and crashes associated with simple sugars. Healthy fats—like those from avocados, olive oil, and nuts—are essential for building cell membranes in the brain and aiding in the absorption of fat-soluble vitamins.

- **Avoid processed food:** Avoiding processed foods and excessive sugar intake is another critical step toward regulating dopamine levels. Highly processed items tend to be laden with refined sugars, unhealthy fats, and additives that can disrupt the delicate balance of neurotransmitters in the brain. Processed foods often cause quick, temporary boosts in dopamine, comparable to the rapid highs and lows experienced with addictive substances. Over time, this can desensitize dopamine receptors and impair natural dopamine production, leading to increased cravings for sugary and processed foods. Consuming these items can also contribute to inflammation and oxidative stress, which are linked to mood disorders such as anxiety and depression (Sutter Health, 2019). Reducing your intake of such foods helps maintain stable mood and energy levels and decreases the likelihood of emotional eating driven by dopamine imbalances.

- **Explore new healthy options:** Experimenting with diverse fruits, vegetables, and whole grains can foster overall well-being and enrich your diet with a wide range of nutrients that support brain health. Introducing variety not only makes meals more enjoyable but also ensures that you receive a comprehensive array of vitamins, minerals, fiber, and antioxidants necessary for optimal brain function. For example, berries are rich in antioxidants known to protect brain cells from oxidative damage and inflammation, while fruits like bananas provide an excellent source of vitamin B_6, aiding neurotransmitter synthesis. Whole grains, including quinoa, buckwheat, and barley, supply a wealth of B vitamins, iron, magnesium, and fiber, all of which help improve cognitive function and stabilize blood sugar levels.

- **Boost the gut-brain connection:** What we eat has a huge impact on how we think and feel. This can be seen through the gut-brain connection. The gut and brain communicate through the vagus nerve, and the gut microbiome produces various neurochemicals that influence brain function, including serotonin, with around 95% being produced in the gut (Sutter Health, 2019). A healthy gut flora therefore supports balanced mood and cognitive function. Eating a diet rich in probiotics—such as yogurt, kefir, sauerkraut, and other fermented foods—can enhance gut health. Eating foods with prebiotic fibers, like garlic, onions, and bananas, is great for your gut health, subsequently having a positive impact on your mental health.

While establishing healthier eating habits, it's important to remain flexible and responsive to your body's unique needs. Everyone's body is different, so individual preferences, intolerances, and lifestyle factors must be considered when changing your diet. Embracing variety and moderation is the key to sustaining long-term dietary changes. You could also consider seeking personalized advice and guidance from a nutritionist or a dietitian who can help you reach your goals.

Replacing Harmful Activities With Productive Ones

Substituting detrimental habits with constructive and fulfilling activities can significantly enhance your quality of life. By focusing on positive changes, you can overcome unhealthy behaviors and develop a more balanced and fulfilling lifestyle. Enriching activities can also be a positive distraction from unhealthy habits you've become dependent on. These are some different ways you can introduce new activities to your daily routine:

- **Identifying triggering situations:** Recognizing environments or emotions that prompt unhealthy behaviors is the first crucial step. A trigger is personalized to you and your life experiences. For some, certain social settings may lead to excessive drinking, while others might find themselves compulsively eating in response to stress. Being able to identify what triggers you takes self-awareness. Keeping a journal to note down situations and feelings that precede indulgent activities can be an effective method of pinpointing specific triggers. This process allows for a greater understanding of what needs to be addressed and changed.

- **Developing coping strategies:** Once triggers are identified, developing coping strategies becomes essential. You want to be able to navigate your triggers so that you don't resort to harmful behaviors. You can achieve this by being more present in each moment, and a technique that can help you achieve this is mindfulness-based stress reduction (MBSR). This technique involves being present in the moment and aware of one's thoughts and feelings without judgment. MBSR can help you recognize when you are about to engage in harmful behavior and choose a healthier alternative instead. Another useful approach is cognitive behavioral therapy, which helps you reframe negative thoughts and develop better responses to triggering situations.

- **Engaging in productive hobbies:** Exploring new interests and passion projects can be a powerful way to replace detrimental habits. Productive hobbies provide a constructive outlet for energy and creativity. A productive activity can be anything that makes you feel fulfilled like nurturing your garden or reading a good book. These activities not only occupy time that might otherwise be spent on harmful behaviors but also offer a sense of accomplishment and purpose. For instance, someone who finds themselves binge-watching TV could substitute this habit with a creative project like writing a book or learning to play the guitar.

- **Investing time in self-improvement:** Self-improvement activities such as reading, learning new skills, or volunteering can also serve as excellent substitutes for unhealthy behaviors. Reading books provides mental stimulation and can increase knowledge on various subjects, offering both entertainment and education. Learning new skills—whether it's cooking a new cuisine, practicing a foreign language, or mastering a new software program—keeps the mind engaged and focused on growth. Volunteering, on the other hand, has the added benefit of contributing to the community and providing a sense of fulfillment and connection with others.

- **Creating a routine:** Establishing a routine can bring structure and predictability to your day, reducing the likelihood of falling back into old habits. Your routine should include activities for both professional and personal fulfillment. Setting aside specific times for meals, physical activity, and leisure can create a balanced schedule that supports overall well-being. Incorporating a daily walk or gym session into your daily schedule can become a healthy habit that replaces time spent on negative activities.

- **Avoiding all-or-nothing thinking:** All-or-nothing thinking can hinder progress. Instead, adopting a flexible mindset that allows for gradual improvement is more sustainable. It's unrealistic to expect perfection immediately. Allowing room for incremental changes and recognizing partial successes helps maintain motivation. For example, if you aim to reduce your screen time, cutting down gradually rather than eliminating it all at once can make the goal more attainable.

Exploring diverse distraction strategies ensures that there are multiple options to turn to when avoiding detrimental habits. This stops you from feeling bored by mundane tasks and activities. Activities such as puzzles, sports, crafting, cooking, or even joining a club or group can be great alternatives. Participating in social activities like book clubs or dance classes can foster connections and provide enjoyable experiences that deter negative behaviors. There are so many enriching alternatives available to you. Find something that works for you.

Key Takeaways for the First Week of Your Dopamine Reset

In this chapter, we have explored several steps to cut out activities that cause dopamine spikes. We started by discussing the importance of reducing technology overstimulation through practices like digital detoxes. Setting specific time limits for device usage and engaging in alternative activities like exercise, mindfulness, and creative pursuits were highlighted as effective ways to manage screen time and promote mental well-being. Don't forget that these strategies can be adapted to help you minimize your engagement in any dopamine-spiking behavior.

Additionally, we examined how balanced nutrition choices can support brain health and help regulate dopamine levels. Avoiding processed foods and incorporating a variety of whole foods into our diets are essential strategies for physical and mental well-being.

By replacing harmful habits with productive ones and developing coping strategies for triggering situations, you can have a successful first week of your detox. Now, let's dive into the next week of this transformative journey, which is all about rewiring your reward system!

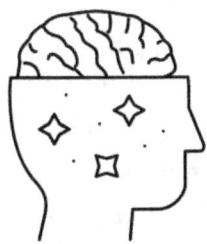

CHAPTER 5

Week 2—Recalibrating Your Reward System

Once you've started to eliminate your harmful addictions successfully, you're ready for week two: recalibrating your reward system. This is an intricate, yet essential process in overcoming technology addiction and other harmful habits. This journey involves shifting how your brain responds to various rewarding activities. However, adjustment isn't always straightforward, and it can come with challenges, particularly when it triggers withdrawal symptoms, which can manifest as intense cravings, irritability, restlessness, and difficulty concentrating. These reactions are your brain's way of coping with the sudden absence of habits you've grown dependent on. Thankfully, there are ways of mitigating these challenges.

In this chapter, we'll delve into recognizing and managing withdrawal symptoms as a pivotal step toward recalibrating your reward system. You'll explore mindfulness practices, like mindful breathing and body scan meditation, that help mitigate these symptoms by promoting self-awareness and relaxation. The chapter aims to equip you with practical tools and insights to navigate this complex transformation, ultimately leading to a healthier and more balanced lifestyle that is consistent even after the 21-day detox.

Understanding and Navigating Withdrawal Symptoms

Adjusting your brain's response to rewarding activities is a challenging but necessary step in breaking free from technology addiction and other unhealthy habits. One of the major hurdles you'll face is dopamine withdrawal symptoms. Recognizing these symptoms can help you better understand what you're experiencing and why it's happening, which is crucial for navigating such a difficult period.

Withdrawal symptoms often manifest as intense cravings, irritability, restlessness, and difficulty focusing. These are your brain's way of reacting to the sudden lack of stimuli it has become accustomed to. For example, if you're used to checking social media frequently, the absence of notifications and constant updates might leave you feeling anxious or unsettled. However, it's important to note that everyone handles their withdrawal from addictive activities differently. It's important for you to observe any behavior or habits that may be out of your character. For example, if you're experiencing random headaches out of nowhere or you're more agitated and restless than usual, it may be your body responding to the absence of your addiction.

How to Handle Your Withdrawal Symptoms

When you're experiencing withdrawal symptoms, you may feel extremely overwhelmed and lost. You might be unsure how to navigate these new behaviors, feelings, and reactions. Using mindfulness practices can be incredibly helpful. Mindfulness is a practice that helps you hone in on your thoughts, feelings, and physical sensations in each moment. This practice can help you acknowledge what's happening within you without feeling overwhelmed by it.

One effective mindfulness technique is mindful breathing. Follow these steps when you feel a craving or any uncomfortable sensation arising:

1. Get comfortable, either seated or lying down.

2. Close your eyes to shut out distractions.

3. Practice some slow and deep breathing. Breathe in through your nose as you mentally count to four, hold this for a beat, and breathe out through your mouth as you count to six.

4. Practice this rhythm of breathing until you feel calmer, both physically and emotionally.

Such a simple exercise can ground you in the present moment and provide relief from stress or anxiety (Gunton, 2024).

Another helpful activity to use when you feel tense is the body scan meditation. By scanning your body from head to toe, you can identify areas that carry tension and stress. Here's how you can practice it:

1. Lie down or sit comfortably, and start by focusing on the top of your head, slowly moving your attention down to your toes.

2. As you observe each part of your body, be aware of where and how you're holding tension in your body.

3. Identify where in your body your withdrawal symptoms are carrying pain and discomfort.

4. Consider why you're experiencing these physical sensations and how you can promote relaxation to avoid them. Getting to the route of the issues mentally can help you to address it physically.

Engaging in this practice daily can build resilience against triggers and lessen the impact of withdrawal symptoms. However, please note that this exercise can be triggering for trauma survivors, and body scan meditations should only be completed if or when they feel safe to you.

Through these mindfulness techniques, withdrawal symptoms can be seen not as hurdles but as opportunities for growth. The discomfort you're experiencing serves as a clear sign that your brain is recalibrating. It's essential to recognize that these symptoms indicate progress rather than failure. Viewing withdrawal through this lens can make the process feel less daunting and more like a necessary step toward positive change.

It's important to understand that recalibrating your reward system won't happen overnight. This process requires gradual effort and consistent commitment. Think of your brain as a muscle that needs training. Just as with physical exercise, mental exercises like mindfulness practices and other coping strategies require consistent practice over time to yield results. Remind yourself that each day you persist, you're strengthening your brain's ability to manage cravings and resist the pull of unhealthy habits.

Additionally, creating a supportive environment can significantly aid in this process. Surround yourself with individuals who understand and support your goals. Whether it's family members, friends, or a support group, having people to talk to can make a big difference. Getting sympathy and encouragement from loved ones who've experienced the same struggles as you can make you feel less alone and more motivated to stay consistent.

Some alternative activities you can practice to get you through your withdrawal symptoms include forms of self-expression, such as journaling or communicating with loved ones, and physical health activities like going for walks or runs. Using a journal to track your progress can also promote accountability and consistency. Writing about your experiences, challenges, and successes can provide insight into your patterns and offer a tangible record of your journey. Reflective journaling allows you to see how far you've come and reaffirms your commitment to change.

Meditation combined with physical exercise, like yoga or tai chi, leverages the mind-body connection to fight off cravings and negative rumination. Research shows that yoga significantly reduces cravings, perceived stress, and anxiety, with effects lasting months post-treatment. This ability to bolster your resilience to triggers makes physical activity an excellent addition to your mindfulness repertoire.

Building Resilience Through Discomfort

Developing resilience in the face of discomfort is an integral part of recalibrating your reward system. This process requires a strong commitment to growth and a willingness to embrace challenges head-on.

Embracing Discomfort

In today's world, it's common to seek immediate gratification and avoid anything that causes unease. But true personal growth often lies just beyond our comfort zones. Think about athletes pushing their limits during training or top students tackling complex subjects; these individuals understand that discomfort is a catalyst for improvement. Although it may be uncomfortable, stepping away from what you're familiar with exposes you to a new world filled with opportunities for growth and learning experiences. Discomfort is not an enemy but a sign that you are challenging yourself and expanding your capabilities.

Consider moments in your life when you have faced discomfort and emerged stronger. Perhaps, it was starting a new job, moving to a different city, or confronting a difficult situation with a friend. These experiences, though uncomfortable at the time, likely contributed to your growth and resilience. By understanding that discomfort is a necessary component of progress, you can begin to view it as a valuable part of your journey rather than something to be avoided.

Shifting Your Mindset

To harness the power of discomfort for personal growth, it's essential to shift your mindset. Viewing discomfort as a temporary state that is essential for development can transform your approach to challenges. Instead of seeing obstacles as unconquerable barriers, you can begin to perceive them as opportunities for learning and growth.

A growth mindset can encourage you to use discipline to fuel your consistency rather than fleeting motivation. This perspective encourages resilience by promoting perseverance in the face of setbacks. Research on growth versus fixed mindsets highlights the importance of how we interpret challenges; a growth mindset fosters resilience, whereas a fixed mindset erects roadblocks (Mandocdoc, 2024).

For example, when learning a new skill, such as playing a musical instrument or speaking a foreign language, initial attempts may be filled with mistakes and frustrations. However, by maintaining a growth mindset, you understand that these early struggles are part of the learning process and that persistence will eventually lead to mastery. This mindset shift makes it easier to remain resilient when faced with discomfort.

Practicing Self-Compassion

While embracing discomfort and adopting a growth mindset are crucial steps, it's equally important to practice self-compassion during challenging times. Self-compassion means being kind and understanding toward yourself, particularly in times of hardship. Studies indicate that adopting a self-compassionate approach can greatly reduce the adverse effects of stress and enhance your ability to cope with challenging situations (*The Power of Mindful Self-Compassion...*, 2024).

Being more self-compassionate can showcase strength in your character. Acknowledge your struggles without fear or judgment. For example, if you're feeling overwhelmed by a difficult task, remind yourself that it's okay to feel this way and that many others have experienced similar challenges. This practice helps create a sense of normalcy around difficult times and reduces feelings of isolation.

Another effective technique is writing a compassionate letter to yourself during times of stress or self-doubt. This method involves expressing empathy, understanding, and encouragement to yourself as you would to a close friend. You deserve to be embraced with love and compassion, especially when navigating such a turbulent journey. Such practices foster a nurturing inner dialogue that can replace negative self-talk and build resilience over time, helping you to avoid the trap of harmful dopamine-seeking cycles.

Developing Endurance

Building long-term resilience requires consistently facing and managing discomfort. This process isn't about making drastic changes overnight but rather developing endurance through small, incremental steps. Just as with physical endurance training, developing mental and emotional resilience takes time and persistence.

Begin by setting achievable goals that gradually push you out of your comfort zone. For example, if socializing with new people in person makes you uncomfortable, start by speaking to one new person at a time and gradually increase the amount of strangers you talk to each day. Progress should always build your confidence, regardless of how small it may seem.

Reward yourself for the endurance you showcase. Acknowledge the milestones you've reached and the challenges you've overcome. These celebrations reinforce your efforts and motivate you to continue facing discomfort with determination.

Practicing Gratitude and Mindfulness

Gratitude and mindfulness are powerful tools that can significantly aid in recalibrating the brain's reward system. By integrating these practices into your daily life, you can encourage positive changes in your brain chemistry, leading to improved mental well-being and a better overall perspective on life.

One effective way to start is by engaging in gratitude exercises. These daily rituals help cultivate appreciation for life's blessings and have been shown to make a substantial impact on emotional health. For example, simple acts like writing down three things you are grateful for each day or expressing thanks to someone who has positively influenced your life can lead to lasting changes in how we perceive the world around us. According to research conducted at UCLA's Mindfulness Awareness Research Center, practicing gratitude on a regular basis can make you happier, as this practice alters the neural structures in your brain (Chowdhury, 2019). This shift toward positivity helps activate the brain's reward center, creating a cycle where gratitude reinforces itself through repeated expression and acknowledgment.

In addition to gratitude exercises, mindful awareness plays a crucial role in rewiring the brain's reward system. It involves being fully present in each moment, savoring all of life's experiences. This form of mindfulness encourages a deeper connection with our surroundings and helps reduce the tendency to seek out short-term pleasures that may not provide lasting happiness. For example, while eating a meal, focusing on the taste, texture, and aroma rather than multitasking can transform a routine activity into a fulfilling experience. Mindfulness helps individuals shift their focus from constant stimulation to appreciating the present moment.

Understanding the impact of gratitude and mindfulness on dopamine levels is essential in recognizing their value in shaping a healthier reward system. When we practice gratitude, our brain releases dopamine, enhancing feelings of joy and contentment (Travers, n.d.). This release creates a positive feedback loop, where the more gratitude we express, the more our brain seeks out situations that elicit these rewarding feelings. Similarly, mindfulness practices also stimulate a slow and sustained release of dopamine, promoting a state of calm satisfaction that counters the anxiety and stress often associated with our fast-paced lives.

To illustrate the transformative power of gratitude and mindfulness, let's unpack the story of John, a busy executive who struggled to find balance in his life: Constantly overwhelmed by work, John decided to incorporate gratitude exercises and mindfulness into his daily routine. Each evening, he spent a few minutes reflecting on three positive aspects of his day and expressing thanks to those who had helped him. He also integrated mindful moments throughout his day, such as by taking deep breaths during stressful meetings or savoring his morning coffee without distractions. Over time, John noticed a significant improvement in his mood and overall sense of fulfillment. He found himself less reactive to stress, more appreciative of small joys, and better able to maintain a positive outlook even amidst challenges.

The benefits of practicing gratitude cannot be overstated. There is so much hope and joy that can be born from expressing your gratitude for people, life, and the world around you. Gratitude enhances empathy and strengthens relationships by encouraging us to value the contributions of others. This fosters a sense of interconnectedness, reducing feelings of isolation and promoting a supportive community environment. Mindfulness, on the other hand, helps improve emotional regulation, allowing us to respond to difficult situations with greater composure and clarity. Together, these practices create a foundation for a more resilient and harmonious life.

Engaging in Creative and Non-Stimulatory Hobbies

The pursuit of activities that shift your focus from excessive stimulation to enriching pursuits is crucial for recalibrating your reward system. By exploring creative outlets, practicing mindful engagement, finding a balance between stimulating and calming activities, and seeking personal fulfillment in non-stimulatory pursuits, we can rewire our brains toward healthier rewards.

Exploring Creative Outlets

Embracing new hobbies that inspire creativity is one of the most effective ways to reduce dependence on dopamine triggers. Creative activities provide a sense of accomplishment and satisfaction without the immediate hit of dopamine that technology and addictive substances offer. For example, picking up a sketchpad and drawing can help divert your focus away from digital screens and onto creating something tangible and meaningful. These activities not only keep the brain engaged but also enhance problem-solving skills and boost overall mental well-being.

On top of that, exploring these healthy and stimulating activities can teach us patience and persistence. Unlike scrolling through social media, creative projects often require time and effort, teaching you to appreciate the process rather than just the end result. As you progress in these activities, you may find yourself experiencing a deeper level of joy that stems from the intrinsic value of creation and self-expression.

Engaging Intentionally

Being fully present while engaging in leisure activities is another powerful way to recalibrate your reward system. Intentional engagement encourages you to savor each experience, whether it's a walk in the park, reading a book, or enjoying a meal. By focusing on the here and now, you allow yourself to break free from the constant need for external stimulation. Practicing intentional activities prevents you from practicing unhealthy habits that are otherwise easy to slip back into. Our digital devices can distract us from being aware of all the greatness that surrounds us each day. Use your spare time to shed light on all the special people and things you get to enjoy every day!

For instance, during your morning coffee, take the time to smell and appreciate the distinct aroma, share gratitude for your cup of coffee, and taste all the complex flavors coffee has to offer. Such mindful engagement transforms an ordinary activity into a rich sensory experience. Regularly practicing mindful engagement can significantly reduce stress and anxiety, as it shifts your focus from the many distractions around you to the soothing simplicity of the present moment.

To successfully integrate mindful awareness into your routine, set aside a few minutes each day for a mindfulness practice. This could be as simple as deep breathing exercises, a short meditation session, or even just sitting quietly and observing your surroundings. Over time, these practices will train your brain to remain calm and focused, enhancing your ability to engage deeply with various activities.

Finding Balance

Striking a balance between stimulating and calming hobbies is essential for a well-rounded lifestyle. While activities that excite and energize you are important, incorporating calmer pursuits can help maintain equilibrium. This balance ensures that you don't become overly dependent on high-stimulation activities to feel fulfilled.

Engaging in physical exercise, for instance, can be both stimulating and calming. As previously mentioned, activities like yoga or tai chi combine movement with mindfulness, promoting physical health while also providing mental relaxation. On the other hand, vigorous exercises like running or playing sports can help release pent-up energy and improve mood by triggering the release of endorphins. Practicing a healthy balance of these activities provides you with the best of both worlds. However, in the early days of your dopamine detox, it's important to engage in more calming activities than stimulating ones.

Another approach to achieving balance is alternating between solitary and social activities. Solitary pursuits, such as reading or journaling, offer introspective time, while social interactions through hobbies like team sports or group classes foster connections and communal enjoyment. A mix of these allows you to enjoy varied experiences without leaning too heavily on one type of activity.

Unearthing Personal Fulfillment

Discovering joy and satisfaction through non-stimulatory activities is the final piece of the puzzle. True fulfillment often comes from activities that nurture your soul rather than provide instant pleasure. Volunteer work, for example, offers immense satisfaction by allowing you to make a positive impact on others' lives. Knitting and making your own clothing can be another fulfilling hobby that's also resourceful and handy to have in your bucket of tricks!

Pursuing intellectual interests can also lead to personal fulfillment. Learning new skills—whether through formal education or self-study—provides long-term rewards by enhancing your knowledge and capabilities. Engaging with literature, art, or music on a deeper level can also enrich your life in ways that go beyond mere entertainment.

As you shift your focus from excessive stimulation to enriching pursuits, you'll likely notice a transformation in your overall mental well-being. The reduced reliance on dopamine triggers will lead to more stable moods and a greater sense of contentment. By embracing creative outlets, practicing mindful engagement, finding balance, and seeking personal fulfillment, you can successfully recalibrate your reward system and pave the way for a healthier, happier life.

Key Takeaways for Week 2: Resetting Your Reward System

Adjusting your brain's response to rewarding activities requires understanding, resilience, and patience. Remember that withdrawal symptoms are expected; these are natural reactions from your brain as it adjusts to a life without the habit it's become so dependent on. By recognizing these symptoms, you can find suitable ways to navigate this challenging period in ways that work for you and your personal detox experience. Practices like mindful breathing and body scan meditation promote relaxation and self-awareness that can help you cope with any seemingly overwhelming withdrawals. They can also present opportunities for personal growth, highlighting the positive changes taking place in your brain.

Patience is crucial in this journey. Recalibrating your reward system is a gradual process that requires consistent effort and commitment. Implementing small lifestyle changes—such as trying out new activities that push you out of your comfort zone—can further support your efforts. Keeping a journal to track your progress and integrating complementary wellness practices like yoga can enhance your resilience and reduce your cravings. Embracing these strategies will help you develop a more balanced and satisfying approach to rewards, contributing to improved mental well-being and a healthier lifestyle. With these tips and strategies, you'll be able to absolutely nail this week of your detox!

Up next, we will explore the third, and final, week of your dopamine reset!

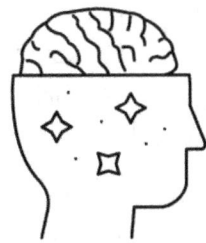

CHAPTER 6
Week 3—Establishing New Habits

You've kicked those addictive habits to the curb, and you're recalibrating your brain's reward system by replacing addictive behaviors with healthier activities. You now want to transform these changes into habits you continue practicing after the 21-day reset. Establishing new habits is fundamental to leading a healthier lifestyle and enhancing mental well-being. Week three zeroes in on creating practices that are not only beneficial but also sustainable for the long haul. It's time to turn changed behavior into healthy habits you stick to in the long run.

The following chapter will explore various methods to monitor habit development and recognize achievements, no matter how insignificant they may appear. You'll learn how to make the most of habits, and you'll even use digital tools to help you reach your goals. This chapter will also address the importance of celebrating milestones and other minor victories, emphasizing their impact on long-term habit formation.

Tracking Progress and Acknowledging Milestones

Forming new habits is a vital part of leading a healthier lifestyle and improving mental well-being. It's crucial to establish practices that are not only healthy but sustainable for the long term. Both elements serve to keep you motivated and committed to your goals. The following points delve into various ways of monitoring your habit development and recognizing achievements, no matter how minor they may seem:

- **Keep a habit journal:** Keeping a habit journal is an effective way to visualize progress and identify patterns in your behavior. By writing down your daily activities, you can see how consistent you are with your new habits. For instance, if your goal is to reduce screen time before bed, jotting down the times you succeed or struggle can reveal triggers that either help or hinder your progress. Over time, you'll be able to discern patterns that might otherwise go unnoticed. This self-awareness is a powerful tool for making adjustments and ensuring that your new habits stick.

- **Download habit-tracking apps:** Utilizing habit-tracking apps can help you use technology productively to monitor your behavioral patterns. These apps offer features to set reminders, mark daily achievements, and even provide visual graphs of your progress. Apps like Habitica and Streaks turn habit tracking into a game, adding an element of fun and competition. Consistently using these tools adds accountability and makes it easier to stay focused on your objectives. Many apps also allow for social sharing, which can further enhance motivation by allowing you to celebrate your small wins with friends or an online community.

- **Share your progress:** On that note, sharing your progress with a friend or joining a support group can provide the extra push you need to stay on track. If you ever find yourself falling off track or being less consistent, check in with your accountability partner to bring you back to consistency. The external validation you receive from someone else can make the journey feel less isolating and more rewarding. Remember, accountability doesn't have to be a rigid process; it can be as simple as sending a weekly update via text message or discussing your progress over a cup of coffee.

- **Reinforce health and fitness milestones:** Fitness milestones are especially significant when developing healthy habits, particularly those involving physical activity. Recognizing improvements in your physical performance can boost your motivation and reinforce your commitment to maintaining a fitness routine. Whether it's running an extra mile, lifting heavier weights, or achieving a new yoga pose, each milestone is a testament to your hard work and dedication. Keeping track of fitness progress can be motivating, as physical achievements might be more tangible and easy to identify compared to your other goals.

- **Acknowledge your progress and reward yourself:** Progress is often made up of small wins, and their importance cannot be overstated. Each small victory propels you forward, creating momentum that keeps you moving toward your ultimate goal. For example, getting up a bit earlier for a walk or choosing a healthier meal option at a restaurant are small steps that gradually lead to more significant changes. Reward yourself with something that brings you joy, so you can feel incentivized to keep going; however, make sure that these rewards are not dopamine-spiking activities or substances that could trigger addictive behaviors again. It's also essential to acknowledge that progress isn't linear. Setbacks will happen, but focusing on small achievements helps maintain a positive outlook.

These strategies form a holistic framework for healthy habit development. Keeping a habit journal allows you to reflect on your journey and make necessary adjustments. Habit-tracking apps provide a modern, interactive way to stay on top of your goals. Accountability systems add a layer of support and encouragement along your dopamine detox journey. Celebrating milestones acknowledges your hard work and reinforces your commitment.

Creating Routines That Support Well-Being

Establishing daily routines that prioritize good, holistic health and sustainable habit formation is crucial for long-term success. By creating structured habits, you can achieve the consistency you need for improved overall health. Let's explore some essential practices to incorporate into your daily life.

Morning and Evening Rituals

Starting the day with positive rituals sets a powerful tone for the hours ahead. A mindful morning routine might begin with a few minutes of meditation, which can ground you and reduce stress. According to Robin Sharma, author of *The 5 a.m. Club*, starting the first hour of your day with healthy activities like exercise, reflection, or journaling can significantly enhance clarity and drive for the day ahead (*Daily Rituals to Boost Health...*, n.d.). For instance, dedicating 20 minutes to strenuous exercise, journaling, meditation, inspirational reading, or setting goals can transform your day.

Equally important are evening rituals. Ending the day with activities like gratitude journaling helps shift your focus toward positivity. Simple acts such as noting three things you're grateful for can foster a sense of abundance and contentment (*Daily Rituals to Boost Health...*, n.d.). Additionally, establishing a calming bedtime routine like disconnecting from electronic devices an hour before sleep can improve sleep quality and help you achieve your digital and dopamine detox goals.

Practice Physical Activity Regularly

Physical activity doesn't have to be strenuous to be beneficial. For example, starting your day with a brisk walk in nature or engaging in a home workout session can energize you and promote a healthier lifestyle. Gentle activities like yoga or stretching can be just as effective for your physical and mental well-being. These practices not only contribute to physical fitness but also offer a form of meditation, helping you connect with your body and reduce stress.

Reflective Journaling

Reflective journaling is a powerful tool for processing thoughts and emotions. By writing down your experiences, feelings, and reflections, you can gain insights into your mental state and identify patterns in your behavior. This practice can be part of both morning and evening routines, providing a sense of clarity and direction. Below are some journal prompts that can help you reflect on your detox journey thus far:

- How have I been handling this detox so far?
- What has been the hardest thing for me to limit or give up during this detox?
- What routines have I put into place to replace the unhealthy ones, and how have they helped me stay consistent?
- How do I see myself pursuing and reinforcing these changes once the 21 days of detox are done?

Use these prompts in your journal, and let them inspire you to create your own prompts for the various phases of resetting your dopamine balance. Answering questions like these in your journal is a great way to identify what kind of space you're in throughout your experience.

In the morning, journaling can serve as a platform for setting intentions for the day. Writing down your goals and aspirations can help keep you focused and motivated. In the evening, it can be a way to reflect on the day's events, acknowledge successes, and process any challenges you face. Regularly reviewing your progress and reflecting on what works and what doesn't can help fine-tune your approach. This reflective practice can lead to more effective and sustainable habit formation that will maintain your neurotransmitter equilibrium.

Building Social Connections and Community Involvement

Social connections play a pivotal role in maintaining healthy habits and overall well-being. Engaging with others not only provides a sense of belonging but also offers opportunities for mutual support and positive influences, which are crucial when stepping away from high-dopamine activities or substances. These are a few ways you can leverage social connections to foster healthier, more sustainable lifestyle changes:

- **Join clubs and groups for support:** Finding support through online or local clubs and groups can connect you with like-minded individuals who share similar interests and challenges. When people engage in activities they enjoy, such as fitness classes, book clubs, or hobby groups, they are more likely to stay committed to their new habits. Being surrounded by individuals who are on the same journey can be highly motivating. It creates a supportive environment where members encourage each other, share tips, and celebrate successes together. For instance, joining a local running group can provide the motivation needed to stick to a regular exercise routine, as members often organize runs, participate in races, and offer encouragement.

- **Volunteer with others:** Participating in volunteer opportunities is another avenue through which social connections can enhance well-being and long-term dopamine regulation. Volunteering not only contributes to a larger community but also fosters a sense of purpose and fulfillment. It allows you to meet new people, build relationships, and develop a support network. Research has shown that volunteering can improve mental health by reducing stress and boosting self-esteem. For example, volunteering at a community garden can promote physical activity while connecting with others who are passionate about gardening and sustainability. The shared experience of working toward a common goal can strengthen social bonds and create lasting friendships.

- **Attend social events:** Attending social events is essential for building relationships outside of typical routines. Social events like community festivals, networking events, or casual gatherings provide opportunities to meet new people and expand one's social circle. These interactions can lead to relationships that guide you along your personal journey toward a healthier life. By diversifying your social interactions, you can learn from others' experiences, gain new perspectives, and find inspiration for your own habit-forming journeys. For instance, attending a wellness workshop might introduce you to new mindfulness practices or nutritional advice, which you can incorporate into your daily life.

These bonds and relationships can be valuable as you navigate adjusting to a mind and body that are no longer dependent on dopamine surges. Moreover, we can all benefit from having a healthy support system that lifts us up when we're feeling worn down and overwhelmed.

The Beauty of Social Connections

The value of social connections transcends simple companionship; it profoundly affects both health and life expectancy. A comprehensive study revealed that robust social bonds can enhance survival rates by 50% (Martino et al., 2017). Strong social support and community involvement correlate with reduced mortality risk, outpacing numerous other cardiovascular disease risk factors. These connections serve as a protective shield against stress, supplying emotional reinforcement and mitigating the effects of adverse situations.

Moreover, social relationships can shape health behaviors through various channels, including emotional support, personal agency, symbolic significance, and societal norms. Emotional support encompasses the nurturing aspects of relationships, such as feeling cherished, valued, and heard (Umberson & Karas Montez, 2010). This can indirectly bolster physical well-being by improving mental health, alleviating stress, and instilling a sense of purpose and meaning. The knowledge that our friends and family are ready to provide encouragement can empower us to navigate through difficult times with ease.

Symbolic meanings attached to social ties also play a significant role in promoting healthy behaviors. Relationships, such as marriage or parenthood, often come with a sense of responsibility to stay healthy and care for one's loved ones (Umberson & Karas Montez, 2010). This sense of duty can drive you to adopt and maintain healthy habits, motivating you to stand strong against any withdrawal symptoms or cravings as you detox from dopamine.

It is important to note, however, that not all social ties are beneficial. Strained, conflict-ridden, or abusive relationships can undermine health and well-being. Therefore, it is crucial to cultivate positive and supportive connections that promote healthy behaviors. Community programs and policies can play a significant role in fostering social connections and reducing social isolation. Initiatives that create public spaces for safe get-togethers promote civic engagement and support stable relationships that enhance individual and community welfare.

Key Takeaways for Week 3 of Your Dopamine Reset

In this chapter, we explored the importance of forming healthier, sustainable habits for long-term well-being. We highlighted various strategies like keeping a habit journal, using habit-tracking apps, and creating accountability systems to monitor progress and keep motivation high. We also learned that recognizing and celebrating small wins—whether through personal milestones or fitness achievements—contributes to building momentum and confidence. These practices are crucial in maintaining a positive outlook and ensuring that new habits become permanent.

To get the most from these strategies, it's essential to integrate them into your daily routine. Consistent tracking, regular check-ins with your support system, and acknowledging each small achievement help solidify new habits. The key is to stay focused on your progress, rather than getting sucked into the negativity of your setbacks. By embedding these approaches into your life, you'll be better equipped to maintain healthy habits and achieve lasting improvements in your mental and physical well-being.

You've completed your 21-day dopamine reset, but the changes don't stop there! Having mental clarity and focus along this journey can help you turn this three-week detox into lasting change. In the next chapter, we will prepare mentally for the continuous journey of self-development and healthy living.

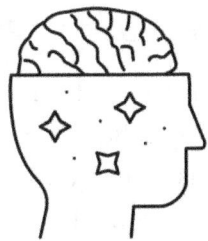

CHAPTER 7
Enhancing Focus and Mental Clarity

Your mentality has a drastic impact on your results when striving for continuous transformation. When you're caught up in unhealthy and dopamine-spiking habits, you aren't engaging your mental focus, as you're most likely going with the motions of your hard-to-resist addictive behavior. Enhancing focus and mental clarity is an essential endeavor to leave bad habits in the past and boost cognitive function.

This chapter delves into practical methods that can sharpen concentration and foster mental resilience, making it easier to navigate the distractions of modern life. By understanding and applying these techniques, you can create a more disciplined and attentive mind that's better equipped to handle daily challenges.

Meditation and Mindfulness Techniques

Meditation and mindfulness have gained significant recognition throughout this book due to their ability to enhance focus and mental clarity. These practices are not just trendy terms but profound tools that can transform cognitive function. Let's delve into how regularly practicing meditation, integrating mindfulness into daily activities, and specific breathing techniques can boost your concentration and overall mental resilience.

Implementing Regular Meditation Practices

We've spoken about using meditation to enhance your mindfulness and minimize impulsive and unhealthy activities, but how can you practice meditation for these desired results? Cultivating a daily meditation routine is one of the most effective ways to enhance cognitive function and clarity. Research has shown that consistent meditation practice helps reduce mental clutter, allowing the brain to focus more efficiently on the tasks at hand. By setting aside even a few minutes daily for focused attention, you can train your mind to become more disciplined and less prone to distraction. Follow these steps to practice meditation successfully:

1. Close your eyes and focus on your breath.
2. Practice deep breathing to calm your mind and your body.
3. As thoughts arise, gently acknowledge them without judgment and return your focus to your breathing. It can be helpful to visualize placing your thoughts on a cloud and watching the wind of your breath blow them away.
4. Over time, increase the duration of these sessions from 5 minutes to 20 or 30 minutes. These increments will help build the discipline needed for extended meditation practices, leading to improved memory and mental clarity (UC Davis Health, 2022).

Mindfulness in Daily Activities

Applying mindfulness to everyday tasks significantly sharpens focus and reduces mental distractions. To be mindful, you must live in the moment, in both mind and body. This might seem simple, but it requires a conscious effort to avoid multitasking and, instead, focus entirely on one task.

We've talked about mindful eating practices, but what are some other daily activities that can be enriched by mindfulness? When walking, notice the sensation of your feet touching the ground, the sound of your footsteps, and the rhythm of your breathing.

Mindfulness can also be incorporated into work routines. Start by dedicating your first hour at the workplace to the most critical task without any interruptions. Mute your phone to avoid the temptation of pinging notifications. This practice—often referred to as "single-tasking"—can dramatically sharpen your focus and productivity throughout the day (National Center for Complementary and Integrative Health, 2022). By practicing mindfulness regularly, these habits become second nature, turning commonplace activities into opportunities for improved mental focus.

Breathing Techniques for Calmness

Practicing specific breathing exercises enhances concentration levels by promoting calmness and reducing stress. Stress is a significant barrier to maintaining focus and mental clarity, as it tends to scatter thoughts and heighten anxiety. Breathing exercises can mitigate these effects by activating the body's natural relaxation response. The following are two valuable breathing techniques to learn:

- **Diaphragmatic breathing:** This breathing technique promotes deep breaths by influencing you to expand your diaphragm as you breathe, rather than your chest. To practice this, lie down or sit comfortably with one hand on your chest and the other on your abdomen. Breathe in slowly through your nose, ensuring your abdomen rises more than your chest. Breathe out your mouth, noticing your abdomen deflating. Repeat this process for 10 breaths, concentrating solely on the movement of your hands and the flow of breath.

- **4-7-8 technique:** Another effective method is the 4-7-8 technique. Inhale gently through your nose until you reach as you mentally count to four, hold your breath for a count of seven, and then exhale through your mouth for a count of eight. This method slows down the heart rate and can quickly induce a state of relaxation, making it easier to focus amid stressful situations.

Combining these practices of regular meditation, mindfulness, and targeted breathing techniques fosters sustained attention and resilience against dopamine dysregulation. The benefits extend beyond improved focus; they also contribute to better emotional regulation, enhanced self-awareness, and reduced anxiety and depression (National Center for Complementary and Integrative Health, 2022).

Cognitive Exercises and Brain Games

Cognitive exercises and brain games are effective tools for enhancing focus and mental clarity. This section will delve into various methods to demonstrate how these tools contribute to improved cognitive functioning.

Puzzles and Memory Challenges

Engaging in puzzles and memory challenges is an excellent way to boost your cognitive function. Activities such as crosswords, sudoku, jigsaw puzzles, and memory card games require concentration, logical reasoning, and pattern recognition. Through regular practice, these activities can significantly enhance mental focus.

Puzzles stimulate multiple areas of the brain, improving not only memory but also spatial awareness and executive function, neurologically reinforcing your ability to resist dopamine desires. For example, solving a crossword puzzle involves retrieving vocabulary from memory, while a jigsaw puzzle requires visual-spatial reasoning.

Implementing puzzles and memory challenges into your routine can be both fun and beneficial. You can start your day with a quick crossword or end it by working on a jigsaw puzzle. Additionally, playing card games that challenge memory, like Concentration or Matching Pairs, can be a social activity that involves friends or family members, making cognitive exercise enjoyable and rewarding.

Alternatively, you can play brain games through online apps. Studies have shown that engaging with brain training apps like Lumosity can result in significant cognitive improvements (Al-Thaqib et al., 2018). One reason behind their efficacy is their ability to adapt to the user's skill level, ensuring that the tasks remain challenging yet achievable, which enhances user engagement and motivation (Kletzel et al., 2021). If you are using digital apps, however, be sure to set boundaries so that you aren't overdoing your screen time.

Critical Thinking Exercises

Practicing critical thinking exercises improves your ability to take on tasks like analyzing information, evaluating evidence, and making reasoned decisions, all of which can be great for a number of reasons. Practices such as debating, discussing complex topics, and engaging in strategic games like chess or checkers can foster critical thinking skills.

Debating, for instance, requires you to construct and defend an argument while also considering counterarguments. This process strengthens your ability to think logically and critically assess information. Similarly, strategy games demand forward-thinking and planning, which can translate to better decision-making skills in real-life situations. This, in turn, improves your impulse control, helping you to avoid slipping back into old, dopamine-seeking patterns.

To integrate critical thinking exercises into your daily life, consider setting aside time to read articles or books that challenge your perspectives. You might wish to join discussion groups or forums where you can engage in meaningful debates and conversations. Additionally, playing strategy-based board games can be a fun way to sharpen your critical thinking abilities.

Implementation Tips

Incorporating cognitive exercises and brain games into your daily routine can seem daunting at first, but with these practical tips it's more than manageable:

- **Start small:** Begin by allocating just 10–15 minutes a day to cognitive exercises. Gradually increase the duration as you become more comfortable with the routine.

- **Mix it up:** Variety is key to keeping your brain engaged. Rotate between different types of activities to ensure a comprehensive cognitive workout.

- **Set goals:** Establishing specific goals for each session can provide motivation and a sense of achievement. For example, aim to complete a certain number of puzzle pieces or reach a new level in a brain training game.

- **Track your progress:** Many brain training apps offer progress-tracking features that allow you to see your improvement over time. Keeping a journal to record your experiences and milestones can also be motivating.

- **Make it Social:** Involve friends or family members in your cognitive exercises. Playing games together or forming a puzzle-solving group can add a social aspect that makes the activities more enjoyable.

- **Integrate exercises into your daily routine:** Find opportunities to incorporate cognitive exercises into your daily life. For instance, you can solve puzzles during your commute, play brain games during lunch breaks, or engage in critical thinking exercises before bedtime.

By following these implementation tips, you can create a sustainable routine that promotes continuous cognitive improvement.

Cognitive Behavioral Therapy for Addiction

Cognitive behavioral therapy (CBT) can help you identify and change harmful patterns that cause or trigger your addictive behaviors. This approach focuses on understanding how thoughts influence feelings and actions. For example, someone struggling with alcohol addiction might think, *I need a drink to relax*. By identifying this thought, they can challenge it and replace it with a healthier perspective, such as, *There are other ways to relax, like going for a walk or talking to a friend.* This shift reduces the urge to drink and promotes healthier coping mechanisms. Some other components of CBT include the following:

- **Identifying triggers:** An important aspect of CBT is identifying triggers that lead to substance use. You may encounter specific situations, people, or emotions that increase your cravings. By mapping out these triggers, you can develop strategies to avoid or cope with them effectively. For example, if a person realizes that being around certain friends makes them want to drink, they can plan to spend time with supportive people instead. This proactive approach empowers you to take control of your recovery.

- **Setting realistic goals:** Through CBT, you learn how to set small, achievable milestones rather than distant, overwhelming objectives. For instance, instead of saying, "I want to quit social media forever," you might aim for one week without using social media. Achieving these smaller goals fosters a sense of accomplishment and builds confidence, making it easier to tackle the next step in your recovery journey.

- **Preventing relapse:** Relapse prevention is another critical component of CBT. You learn to identify warning signs of potential relapse and develop a plan to address them. This might include creating a list of coping strategies or seeking support from friends and family during challenging times. By preparing for setbacks, you can respond constructively and avoid falling back into old habits.

- **Encouraging mindfulness:** In addition, CBT encourages mindfulness practices. This self-awareness can significantly reduce the likelihood of impulsive actions driven by cravings. By practicing mindfulness, you can observe cravings as temporary events rather than a part of your being that defines you. This separation allows you to choose your responses more consciously.

How CBT Works

The structure of dopamine detox-focused CBT often includes scheduled sessions with a therapist who specializes in addiction treatment. These sessions provide a safe space for you to explore your thoughts and feelings openly. The therapist will guide the conversation, helping you navigate the complexities of your addiction. Attending regularly helps maintain accountability and progress toward recovery goals, and homework assignments are commonly included to reinforce learning between sessions.

Cognitive distortions, or inaccurate thought patterns, are another area of focus in CBT. Many people with addiction problems tend to engage in all-or-nothing thinking. For example, after one slip-up, you may think, *I've failed completely, so I might as well give up*. This type of thinking can, of course, be extremely detrimental. CBT teaches clients to recognize these thoughts and reframe them into more balanced views, enabling them to maintain progress even after setbacks.

Building self-esteem is equally important in CBT for addiction. Individuals struggling with addiction often suffer from low self-worth, believing they are unworthy of recovery. Through positive reinforcement and focusing on personal strengths, CBT can help you cultivate a more positive self-image. This newfound confidence can motivate you to pursue healthier lifestyle choices and relationships away from your addictive behavior.

CBT also incorporates strategies for managing cravings. Techniques such as distraction, deep breathing, or engaging in enjoyable activities can offer relief when cravings strike. Learning to implement these strategies and being supported as you practice them can lessen the intensity of cravings and increase your capacity to resist temptations. Over time, the practice of using these techniques can lead to lasting changes in your habits and thought patterns.

Furthermore, CBT teaches problem-solving skills. You learn to approach challenges rather than avoid them. This active engagement helps build resilience and fosters the ability to tackle issues as they arise.

By cultivating these skills, you can navigate life's difficulties without resorting to substances.

CBT is also adaptable, making it suitable for various forms of addiction, including substance abuse, and compulsive behaviors like gambling, binge spending, overconsumption of media, or overeating. Each person's experience is unique. CBT is special as it addresses your specific needs and circumstances. This flexibility allows for a personalized treatment approach that can resonate more deeply.

Ultimately, the goal of CBT in addiction recovery is to equip you with the tools you need to lead a fulfilling, substance-free life. By addressing underlying thought patterns, building coping strategies, and fostering self-awareness, CBT can create lasting behavioral changes. As you continue to practice these skills, you cultivate a healthier relationship with yourself and the world around you.

Support groups often complement CBT, offering a space for individuals to share their journeys. This community support reinforces the lessons learned in therapy, providing encouragement and additional resources.

As people progress through a CBT program, they often experience a shift in identity. You are likely to start viewing yourself not as an addict but as an individual on a journey of recovery. This transformation is essential for sustaining change. Your new identity can lead to healthier choices, improved relationships, and a more meaningful life.

Through continued practice and commitment to the principles of CBT, you can build a foundation for long-term recovery. The skills developed in therapy extend beyond addiction management; they can also enhance various aspects of life, including work, parenting, and personal relationships.

The Impact of Sleep on Focus

The importance of sleep in maintaining focus and mental clarity cannot be overstated. Our modern lifestyles can often make it challenging to get a good night's sleep, but understanding the difference between quality and quantity can help improve cognitive function and dopamine regulation. Here are some valuable tips that can help you understand the value of sleep and how you can boost your focus through improved sleep quality:

- **Quality versus quantity of Sleep:** While many people emphasize the number of hours spent asleep, the quality of those hours is equally crucial. Quality sleep is characterized by uninterrupted, deep rest that leaves you feeling refreshed upon waking. Poor quality sleep, even if abundant in hours, can lead to grogginess and impaired cognitive function. Research has shown that during high-quality sleep, the brain undergoes essential processes like memory consolidation and toxin removal, which are vital for cognitive health (Wein, 2021). Ensuring that each hour of sleep is effective can have a significant impact on your ability to focus and think clearly throughout the day.

- **Sleep hygiene practices:** Good sleep hygiene is fundamental to achieving restful and restorative sleep, which subsequently boosts focus and mental sharpness. Simple practices such as maintaining a consistent sleep schedule, creating a calming bedtime routine, and optimizing your sleep environment can make a big difference. For instance, keeping the bedroom dark, cool, and quiet fosters better sleep. Don't forget to limit your exposure to screens before you sleep. It's also helpful to avoid caffeine and heavy meals before you go to bed to improve your quality of sleep. Adopting these habits helps ensure that the sleep you get is truly beneficial, setting the stage for better cognitive performance (Vyas, 2023).

- **Napping for a cognitive boost:** Strategic napping can provide a significant cognitive boost, especially when one experiences afternoon slumps. Short naps, ideally lasting 10–20 minutes, can enhance alertness and performance without interfering with nighttime sleep. Longer naps may lead to sleep inertia—a state of grogginess that can be counterproductive. Naps can help with memory consolidation and recharging the brain. In fact, studies suggest that a quick nap can improve learning efficiency and problem-solving skills. Incorporating well-timed naps into your routine can be a powerful tool for maintaining peak mental performance throughout the day.

- **Lifestyle integration:** Prioritizing sleep should be seen as an integral part of a healthy lifestyle rather than an optional luxury. Consistent improvements in mental clarity are observed when sleep is given due importance. This means actively making time for sleep despite busy schedules and recognizing its role in overall well-being. For instance, regular physical activity and balanced nutrition support better sleep patterns and a holistic approach to health.

Understanding that sleep influences not only cognitive functions but also emotional stability and physical health can motivate you to integrate these sleep-friendly habits into your daily routine.

How to Gain Mental Clarity and Focus During a Detox

In this chapter, we explored various strategies to enhance concentration and cognitive function, focusing on meditation, mindfulness, and effective breathing techniques. Regular meditation can significantly clear mental clutter, while mindfulness practices encourage full engagement in everyday tasks to sharpen focus. Additionally, specific breathing exercises help reduce stress and promote a calm state of mind, further aiding concentration.

Integrating these practices into your daily routine can lead to noticeable improvements in mental clarity and emotional welfare. By dedicating a few minutes each day to these activities, you can build resilience against distractions and maintain a sharp, focused mind. These habits not only boost cognitive performance but also contribute to a healthier, more balanced lifestyle.

There's so much more to learn about dopamine that can help you master it in your daily life. In the next chapter, we will discuss some valuable insights about dopamine that can help you balance it in your life in the long term.

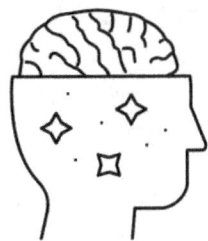

CHAPTER 8
Scientific Insights Into Dopamine and Addiction

Dopamine and addiction are intricate and scientific topics that are constantly being researched and studied. Understanding as much as we can about our reward system and its influence on our behaviors can guide us to better decision-making processes. This chapter delves into the more detailed science behind this vital neurotransmitter, exploring its interaction with other chemicals in our brains and how it impacts our actions.

In this chapter, we'll explore the ways dopamine collaborates with other neurotransmitters like serotonin to create feelings of pleasure and satisfaction. The connection between dopamine and addictive behaviors will also be discussed, uncovering why overcoming addiction requires more than just willpower. Additionally, the concept of genetics and its impact on dopamine and addiction will be uncovered. Learning about the insights that dopamine research has provided helps us understand more about addiction and how to overcome it, as well as empowering us to take a self-compassionate approach to detoxing.

The Neuroscience Dopamine Regulation

We've discussed dopamine, the reward system, and how this neurotransmitter and neural structure work hand-in-hand, but there are some of the intricacies behind this neuroscience. By examining dopamine's physiological role in reward responses, motivation, and reinforcement, we can better comprehend why certain behaviors become habitual and what makes them difficult to change.

Neuroplasticity allows our brains to adapt to new situations, learn from experiences, and recover from injuries. In the context of habits, neuroplasticity means that repeated behaviors can strengthen specific neural pathways, making these behaviors more automatic over time. This plasticity not only facilitates habit formation but also provides opportunities for change. For instance, breaking a bad habit involves weakening the established neural connections while simultaneously creating and reinforcing new, healthier pathways. This process requires consistent effort and engagement in alternative behaviors to rewire the brain effectively.

Therefore, although neuroplasticity can be used to form toxic habits that lead to addiction, it can also result in positive habits when navigated correctly. This is why knowledge about dopamine is important, as it allows you to use this aspect of your own brain to your advantage. You can use this information to make calculated decisions that benefit you in the long term rather than in the moment.

Dopamine plays a central role in shaping our behaviors through its interactions with other neurotransmitters, its influence on motivation and reinforcement, and its involvement in the reward pathway linked to addiction. But neuroplasticity provides hope and strategies for changing undesirable habits by leveraging the brain's inherent ability to adapt and rewire itself. Understanding these mechanisms is crucial for anyone looking to break free from technology addiction or other unhealthy habits to improve mental well-being and lead a healthier lifestyle. Whether it's by adopting new routines, setting up healthy reward systems, or seeking professional help, knowing how dopamine functions can empower you to take control of your habits and ultimately your life.

The Role of Genetics in Addiction

Understanding how genetic factors contribute to addiction and dopamine regulation is complex but crucial. The interplay between our genes and the environment profoundly influences our behaviors, including those related to addiction and dopamine signaling. Understanding these influential relationships can help you navigate your addiction.

Genetic variations play a significant role in determining an individual's susceptibility to addiction by affecting dopamine receptors and transporters. Variations in genes coding for dopamine receptors, such as the DRD2 gene, can impact how individuals respond to rewards and stresses. These variations may result in some people having a heightened pleasure response from addictive substances, making them more vulnerable to developing addictive behaviors.

Researchers have identified specific single-nucleotide polymorphisms (SNPs) that correlate strongly with overall addiction susceptibility. In a comprehensive investigation involving over one million participants, scientists discovered 19 distinct SNPs connected to general addiction risk and 47 SNPs linked to particular substance use disorders among people of European descent (National Institute on Drug Abuse, 2023). This highlights the influence of genetic variations on dopamine signaling and, in turn, the likelihood of developing addiction.

Environmental Factors Influencing Dopamine

Environmental factors also exert a considerable influence on gene expression related to dopamine. The study of epigenetics examines how gene expression can be modified by external factors without changing the DNA code itself, illustrating the dynamic interaction between our environment and genetic activity. Stressors, trauma, and exposure to certain substances can lead to epigenetic modifications that affect dopamine-related pathways. For example, early-life stress has been shown to cause lasting changes in the genes regulating dopamine, which can increase vulnerability to addictions later in life.

One notable aspect of this relationship is the phenomenon known as gene-environment interaction, where the effect of environmental exposure on behavior is influenced by an individual's genetic makeup. Certain genetic variants may amplify the impact of environmental stressors, making those carrying these variants more prone to addiction when exposed to stressful or traumatic experiences. For example, monoamine oxidase A (MAOA) and the serotonin transporter, SLC6A4, have been implicated in individual differences in stress resilience and subsequent addiction risk (Ducci & Goldman, 2012).

Research has also delved into the heritability of addictive behaviors linked to dopamine signaling. Family and twin studies have consistently demonstrated that there is a substantial genetic component to addiction. Twin studies, in particular, have shown that identical twins—who, of course, share all their genes—are more likely than fraternal twins to both develop addiction if one twin is addicted, suggesting a strong genetic influence (National Institute on Drug Abuse, 2023).

The interaction between genetics, the environment, and addiction susceptibility is intricate and multifaceted. It's not just about having a set of "addiction genes." Instead, it's how these genes interact with environmental exposures and individual experiences that ultimately determine addiction risk. Lifestyle choices—such as diet, level of physical activity, and stress management—can also influence dopamine-related pathways through epigenetic mechanisms.

When combined with adverse environmental factors, genetic predispositions can create a fertile ground for addiction. An individual with a genetic makeup that makes their dopamine system highly sensitive might not necessarily develop an addiction unless exposed to high levels of stress, trauma, or addictive substances. Conversely, someone with a less sensitive dopamine system might need higher doses of an addictive substance to experience the same pleasure, potentially leading to higher usage and eventual addiction.

Chronic stress also has a prominent impact on dopamine gene expression. It can lead to increased release of cortisol—a stress hormone that interacts with dopamine pathways. Prolonged exposure to high cortisol levels can alter how dopamine is regulated, increasing the risk of addiction. Studies have shown that individuals exposed to chronic stressors are more likely to engage in substance use as a coping mechanism, particularly if they carry genetic variants that make their dopamine system more reactive to stress.

Understanding intermediate phenotypes—hereditary traits associated with disease risk—can shed light on how genetic and environmental factors converge. For example, a low response to alcohol is a trait influenced by genetic variations and an intermediate phenotype that could indicate a higher risk of developing alcoholism. By identifying these traits, researchers can better understand the pathways leading to addiction and develop targeted interventions.

This nuanced understanding of the relationship between genetic factors and addiction does not imply determinism. Having a genetic predisposition does not guarantee addiction; it merely increases a person's susceptibility. Early intervention, supportive environments, and healthy lifestyle choices can mitigate these risks. Personalized approaches to prevention and treatment, tailored to your unique genetic and environmental background, can help you practice more effective management of your addiction.

Future Directions in Dopamine Research

We are constantly learning new things about ourselves through research. Scientists practice frequent studies to discover how our bodies work and why we behave in the ways we do. Dopamine has only been researched for about 50 years, so there's still much more for us to learn. The future of dopamine research is expansive and exciting. Here are some aspects of exploration we can expect to find:

- **Genetic studies:** Research into the genetics behind dopamine receptors and transporters is ongoing, with the potential to uncover how individual differences in dopamine function contribute to diverse behaviors and susceptibility to mental health disorders.

- **Neuroimaging advances:** Cutting-edge neuroimaging techniques will allow scientists to map dopamine pathways in greater detail than ever before, providing new insights into its role in health, habits, and disease.

- **Targeted therapies:** Advances in understanding dopamine's role in various conditions will lead to more targeted therapies. For example, new drugs aimed at modulating specific dopamine pathways may offer better treatment outcomes for disorders like schizophrenia, depression, and Parkinson's disease.

Understanding the neurobiology of addiction through dopamine pathways could further reveal why some individuals are more susceptible to addictive behaviors than others. Genetic variations that affect dopamine receptors may help explain these differences. We've already learned a lot about dopamine through genetic studies, and we can expect to discover even more as research continues.

Recent studies using neuroimaging techniques have shown that individuals struggling with addiction have altered dopamine signaling, especially in areas of the brain responsible for decision-making and impulse control. When an individual engages in behavior that stimulates the release of dopamine, such as using drugs or gambling, it creates a strong sense of pleasure. Over time, repeated exposure can lead to changes in the brain that enhance the drive to seek out these rewarding experiences, often at the expense of other interests and responsibilities. This cycle of craving and use reinforces itself, making recovery challenging.

Targeting the neural circuits involved in addiction is a promising area for treatment development. Researchers are exploring pharmacological interventions that can help normalize dopamine activity in the brain. For instance, medications that stabilize or modulate dopamine release may reduce cravings and withdrawal symptoms, providing essential physiological support for individuals in recovery. Additionally, behavioral therapies designed to help patients re-engage with healthy sources of reward can complement these pharmacological approaches, creating a more comprehensive treatment plan.

Current innovations are also focusing on personalized medicine in addiction treatment. By considering each individual's genetic makeup and specific dopamine pathway dysfunctions, therapies can be tailored to maximize effectiveness. Understanding how distinct polydrug use patterns affect dopamine signaling can inform treatment strategies. Furthermore, advancements in technology are allowing researchers to monitor brain activity and behavior in real time, leading to greater insights into addiction processes. This data-driven approach holds the potential to see which treatments work best for specific individuals and which factors may predict treatment response.

Additionally, research on dopamine's involvement in behavioral addiction is gaining traction. These forms of addiction may not involve substances, but they still rely heavily on dopamine's reward pathways. Modern technology amplifies these effects, leading to compulsive behaviors that can disrupt everyday life. Understanding how dopamine influences these behaviors can inform new preventative measures and treatment options. This area remains particularly relevant for younger generations who are often more vulnerable to these emerging forms of addiction.

The link between dopamine and stress also plays a significant role in addiction research. Chronic stress can alter dopamine signaling, which may increase vulnerability to substance use as individuals seek relief or escape. Studies are investigating how stress-management techniques, combined with addiction treatments, can help restore balance to the dopamine system and support recovery. Reducing stress could mitigate the impacts on dopamine activity, ultimately aiding in the prevention of relapse.

As more is understood about the complex interactions between dopamine and addiction, researchers are passionate about sharing their findings with the public. Awareness campaigns are being launched to educate communities about the science of addiction and the importance of seeking help. By demystifying the role of dopamine in problematic behaviors, these efforts may reduce stigma and encourage individuals to seek treatment sooner.

Innovative approaches in neuroscience, such as optogenetics, are beginning to shed light on the precise mechanisms by which dopamine influences addiction pathways. Researchers are using these techniques to activate or inhibit specific dopamine circuits in animal models, allowing for a better understanding of how altering these pathways can affect behavior. This type of research could pave the way for advanced treatment modalities that specifically target the dopamine system at a very granular level.

Understanding the interplay between dopamine, mental health, and addiction is crucial for developing holistic treatment strategies. When struggling with both addiction and mental health issues, it's crucial to receive professional attention and guidance. Integrated care—which combines addiction treatment with mental health services—has shown promise in improving outcomes. Ongoing research will help refine these integrated models, ensuring that patients receive comprehensive support tailored to their unique needs.

The future of dopamine research holds immense potential for groundbreaking discoveries. As scientists uncover the nuances of how dopamine influences various behaviors and conditions, new avenues for effective treatments will emerge. This work not only highlights the importance of neuroscience but also emphasizes the need for interdisciplinary collaboration among researchers, clinicians, and policymakers. In pursuing better understanding and treatment of dopamine-related disorders, society moves closer to addressing these pressing public health challenges.

Clinical trials focusing on dopamine-targeted therapies are already underway, demonstrating the rapid progress being made in this field. These trials aim to provide further evidence supporting the efficacy of novel interventions, potentially leading to new approved treatment options. Engaging with patients throughout the research process could also yield valuable insights, ensuring that studies remain relevant to those affected by addiction.

Finally, ethical considerations around dopamine research are becoming increasingly important as new technologies are developed. Questions regarding consent, privacy, and the implications of genetic testing for addiction susceptibility arise. Researchers and ethicists must collaborate to establish guidelines that protect individuals while advancing the field. Open dialogue and transparency in research practices will be essential in fostering trust and promoting engagement in future studies.

The Path to Overcoming Addiction

Addiction can be a tough battle for many. As we have seen, it involves both biological and environmental factors, meaning that some people might be more likely to struggle with it due to their genes or their experiences. If someone in your family has dealt with addiction, you might feel its pull more strongly. But regardless of your family history, addiction can affect the brain's reward system by altering your levels of dopamine. This disruption can lead to a cycle of seeking that pleasure through the substance or habit. Though addictive behaviors can be so challenging to walk away from, there is a way out, regardless of how big or small your habit may seem. By using the resources and strategies available to you, you can break free from unhealthy routines that are holding you back in your life.

Resources for Overcoming Digital Addiction

As previously discussed, digital addiction is becoming increasingly common in our tech-driven world. People often find themselves compulsively checking their phones, scrolling through social media, or playing video games for endless hours. To tackle digital addiction, use the strategies mentioned in early chapters, such as setting screen-time limits and establishing tech-free zones. Additionally, you can embark on a tech-free journey with a group of friends. Challenge yourselves by engaging in outdoor activities and new adventures with no involvement of digital devices. By consciously making an effort to reduce digital consumption, you can redirect your focus to more fulfilling and productive pursuits.

Resources for Overcoming Food Addiction

Food addiction can also be a significant hurdle for many people. It generally involves an obsession with eating or an inability to control food consumption. To tackle this issue effectively, consider establishing a weekly meal plan. By organizing your meals in advance, you can curb impulsive eating tendencies and cultivate healthier dietary habits. Incorporate a diverse selection of fruits, vegetables, whole grains, lean proteins, and unsaturated fats to achieve well-rounded nutrition. Additionally, becoming part of a support group can offer motivation as you face these obstacles. Exchanging stories and learning from others can nurture a strong sense of belonging that combats dopamine dependence.

Resources for Overcoming Substance Addiction

When it comes to addiction to substances, such as alcohol or drugs, it is essential to seek professional help. Acknowledging your addiction means you can take actionable steps to recover. This acknowledgment can be daunting, but it is crucial for starting the recovery process. Therapy is a critical part of healing and recovery. Speaking with a trained counselor or therapist can help you work through underlying issues and develop coping strategies. Consider exploring local treatment centers or support groups like Alcoholics Anonymous (AA) or Narcotics Anonymous (NA), where you can connect with individuals who have similar experiences.

Substance detoxification is often an initial step in overcoming this form of addiction. This process can be uncomfortable and requires medical supervision, especially if withdrawal symptoms arise. It's important to prioritize your physical health while you're recovering. Seeking medical advice and following a healthcare professional's guidance can ensure that you are taking the right steps to heal your body safely.

Practicing healthy habits can also facilitate recovery. Developing a solid support network of friends and family can provide encouragement when you face challenges. Moreover, as touched on previously, engaging in physical activities such as jogging, yoga, or team sports can also boost your mood while keeping you occupied. Finding new hobbies to distract you from your cravings is another strategy that shouldn't be overlooked.

Focusing on Mental Health

Improving your mental health can drastically impact the way you perceive your behaviors and addiction. Many people struggle with feelings of anxiety, depression, or low self-esteem during their recovery process. Mindfulness and stress-relieving activities are important when your mental health is being negatively impacted. It's also advisable to seek professional treatment options, like CBT, which can help address negative thinking patterns and improve your coping strategies.

Through engaging with these various strategies and resources, overcoming addiction is possible. It's a long road, but with determination and the right support and methods, anyone can find their way to a healthier lifestyle.

Key Insights Into the Science Behind Dopamine and Addiction

Throughout this chapter, we have explored the intricate role that dopamine plays in shaping our behaviors and forming habits. We delved into what we know about dopamine now and what insights we might look forward to discovering in the future. Understanding the mechanisms behind dopamine dependence offers valuable knowledge about why some of our habits are so difficult to break and points to potential strategies for behavioral change.

Recognizing the connection between dopamine and habit formation emphasizes the importance of neuroplasticity—the brain's ability to reorganize itself and form new neural connections. This adaptability means that while habits can become deeply ingrained over time, they are not set in stone. By consistently engaging in alternative, healthier behaviors and making use of the resources available to you, it is possible to rewire your brain and establish new patterns.

Leveraging the science of dopamine can empower you to take control of your habits, fostering a path toward an improved and more fulfilling lifestyle. The goal is to make these changes a long-lasting habit that helps you live a higher quality of life. In the next chapter, we will discuss how you can use your knowledge of dopamine to successfully stick to this transformation beyond the 21-day detox.

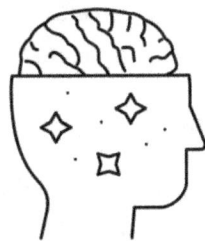

CHAPTER 9
Maintaining Balance Post-Detox

The changes that you make to your lifestyle shouldn't just be a temporary fix but rather a long-term transformation. Maintaining dopamine balance post-detox is essential for achieving these long-lasting results and avoiding relapse after completing *The 21-day Dopamine Reset* detox. The momentum gained during the detox period must be sustained through consistent strategies that reinforce new habits and counter potential setbacks.

In this chapter, we will explore various techniques to keep you on track after detox. You will learn about the importance of routine check-ins and how they can help you reflect on your progress and make necessary adjustments. Additionally, we will discuss the value of accountability partners in supporting your efforts and offering feedback. By focusing on these strategies, this chapter aims to equip you with practical tools and insights to maintain balance and achieve lasting well-being.

Monitoring and Adjusting Post-Detox Habits

After the detox, the real work comes into play. Working on building long-lasting healthy habits and practicing the discipline to stick to them showcases true dedication to personal growth and fulfillment. The following tips will guide you as you adjust to a new lifestyle post-detox.

Establishing a Routine for Check-Ins

Maintaining the momentum gained during the detox period is crucial for long-term success. Regularly check in on your routine, goals, and expectations to ensure you're staying aligned with your vision. These reflection sessions serve as opportunities to pause, assess, and make necessary adjustments to your habits.

Regular check-ins can be scheduled weekly or bi-weekly, depending on what works best for you. Ask yourself questions such as, "Have I been consistent with my new habits?" and "Are there any triggers that have led me to revert to old behaviors?" Reflecting on these questions helps you stay conscious of your actions and aware of any areas needing improvement.

Additionally, consider integrating goal-setting into your check-in routine. Setting clear, immediate objectives enables you to sustain your concentration and drive. These objectives should be practical and attainable within a specified period. For instance, if one of your goals is to reduce screen time, set an incremental target like limiting it by 30 minutes each week until you reach your desired level.

Make sure to keep a journal or log in which you document your reflections and goals during each check-in session. Writing things down not only solidifies your commitment but also provides a record to track your journey and recognize your milestones.

Utilizing Habit-Tracking Tools

To sustain the benefits achieved during your detox, leveraging habit-tracking tools can be immensely helpful. These tools—such as journals, calendars, or apps—allow you to monitor your progress consistently and ensure you're staying on track.

Digital habit-tracking apps are particularly useful due to their convenience and advanced features. However, if you'd like to steer away from the use of digital devices, you can take the more tangible approach by using a physical journal or planner to track your habits. Write down your daily habits, and mark them off as you complete each one each day. The act of physically checking off a task can be highly satisfying and motivating.

Choose the tool that aligns best with your lifestyle and preferences. Whether digital or analog, the key is to use it consistently and make it part of your daily routine.

Seeking Continuous Help From Accountability Partners

Another powerful strategy for maintaining balance post-detox is seeking help from your accountability partners. We've touched on accountability partners previously, but now, it's time to look at how you can go about forming these important relationships. Making this commitment with others who share similar goals can provide the support, encouragement, and feedback needed to stay committed to your new habits.

Potential accountability partners can be anyone who is also striving for self-improvement and better habits. This might include your friends, family members, or colleagues. Ask someone who is open to this journey if they would like to make the big jump together. Discuss strategies and guidelines you can follow so that you're both on the same page. Keeping clear communication throughout this process ensures that you avoid miscommunications and can have healthy boundaries while you hold each other accountable. Be sure to regularly check in with each other, share your progress, and discuss any challenges you're facing. This mutual support system can significantly boost your motivation and resilience during tougher times.

Joining support groups, either online or in person, is another excellent way to find accountability partners. Many communities focus on various aspects of habit change, from reducing tech use to improving mental well-being. Being part of such a community offers a sense of belonging and shared purpose, which can be incredibly uplifting.

For those who prefer a more structured approach, hiring an accountability coach can be beneficial. Coaches offer professional guidance and hold you accountable through regular check-ins and personalized feedback. Apps like GoalsWon combine coaching with goal tracking, making it easier to stay on course (*23 Apps That Will Keep You Accountable*, 2023).

Consistency in Monitoring

Consistency is a cornerstone of maintaining progress after a detox. In addition to establishing a regular schedule for habit reviews, it's important to gather sufficient data to analyze during these check-ins. Monitoring your adherence to new, healthy behaviors ensures sustained progress and helps prevent relapse into old patterns.

Set aside specific times during the day dedicated solely to recording your habits. This could be part of a gratitude practice every evening or a routine part of how you motivate yourself in the morning; choose a time that fits seamlessly into your routine. Consistency in scheduling this time to monitor your progress reinforces their importance and makes them a habitual part of your life.

During these sessions, evaluate your adherence to the established habits. Are there any areas where you've slipped? If so, identify the reasons and devise strategies to address them. Consistent monitoring allows for immediate corrective action, ensuring that small lapses don't snowball into significant setbacks before your larger check-in.

Consistently monitoring your progress and checking in with your advancement toward your short- and long-term goals ensures that you're always aligned with your progress expectations. It serves as a constant reminder of the progress you've made and the effort required to maintain it.

Establishing Long-Term Plans

While short-term goals are essential, developing a long-term plan for habit maintenance is equally critical. Long-term planning involves setting broader objectives and defining the steps needed to achieve them over an extended period.

Consider what you want to achieve in six months, a year, or even five years. Make your goals concise and small. For example, if your ultimate goal is to lead a healthier lifestyle, break it down into actionable steps like exercising regularly, eating balanced meals, and maintaining a healthy sleep schedule.

Having a vision for the future provides direction and motivation, making it easier to stay disciplined in your daily habits. It also allows for flexibility and adaptation as you grow and evolve in your journey.

Regularly review and adjust your long-term plans to reflect any changes in your circumstances or aspirations. Life is dynamic, and being adaptable while staying committed to your overarching goals is key to sustained progress.

Staying Motivated and Rewarding Yourself

Maintaining new habits can sometimes feel challenging, especially after the initial enthusiasm runs dry. To counter this, find ways to stay motivated and reward yourself for your efforts.

Identify what makes you feel motivated to keep going. It could be the satisfaction of ticking off tasks, seeing visual progress in a habit tracker, or receiving positive feedback from accountability partners. Leverage these motivators to keep your spirits high and your drive intact. Don't forget to reward yourself for achievements, no matter how small they may seem!

Setting up a rewards system tied to your habits can also be effective. For instance, if you stick to your habit for an entire month, reward yourself with something special. This creates a positive feedback loop that encourages continued adherence to your new routines, while also fostering a healthy relationship with dopamine that is based on consistency rather than craving.

Continual Self-Assessment and Reflections

In maintaining long-term results post-detox, many people find that self-assessment and reflection are critical tools. These practices are particularly important after undergoing a *21-day Dopamine Reset* detox, as they help to solidify the behavioral changes made during the initial detox period, thus preventing relapse. The following components of long-lasting transformation can help you to reflect and adapt each day:

- **Heightened awareness:** Self-reflection practices play a significant role in developing real-time self-awareness. By incorporating reflection into your daily routine, you can evaluate your thoughts and actions more clearly. This practice involves being present in the moment and observing your internal experiences without judgment. Research indicates that mindfulness enhances cognitive control, attentional regulation, and emotional stability (Schuman-Olivier et al., 2020). For example, if you were to set aside a few minutes each day for mindful breathing or body scans, you would become significantly more aware of your mental states and behavioral patterns. This heightened awareness can aid in identifying negative thoughts and impulses before they escalate into actions, thus fostering healthier habits.

- **Identifying triggers:** Improved self-awareness can make it easier for you to identify triggers and patterns that could lead to relapse. Many people relapse not because they lack willpower, but because they're unaware of the triggers that lead them back to old habits. Recognizing these triggers requires careful observation and reflection on past behaviors. It might be useful to keep a journal to note situations, emotions, or environments that spark urges to revert to previous habits. Once these triggers are identified, strategies can be devised to address them effectively. This might involve altering your environment, developing new coping mechanisms, or learning to navigate high-risk situations through preparation and planning.

- **Setting goals regularly:** Regular goal setting is another vital component of maintaining balance after detox. Setting new targets helps to continue personal growth and development. Goals provide direction and motivation, keeping you focused on your journey toward better mental well-being. It's beneficial to create a vision board or write down goals to visualize progress continually. Remember to break down larger objectives into smaller, manageable tasks so that it's easier to achieve and maintain long-term success.

- **Regular self-assessments:** As we have seen above, evaluating progress continuously is equally necessary. Regular assessments allow you to see how far you've come and what areas still need improvement. This ongoing evaluation keeps motivation high and provides a sense of accomplishment. Simple methods such as weekly check-ins or monthly reviews can be immensely beneficial. You might ask yourself questions like, "What has improved since starting this journey?" or "What challenges have I faced, and how did I overcome them?" This reflection not only highlights successes but also identifies areas where additional effort is needed.

- **Being proactive:** Addressing your triggers requires a proactive approach. Strategies should be adapted to you and your personal experience. For example, if certain apps or websites are encouraging problematic dopamine-seeking patterns, uninstalling them or setting usage limits can help. Additionally, developing more broad and accessible coping strategies—such as deep breathing exercises or engaging in distracting activities—can mitigate the urge to relapse. Cognitive behavioral techniques such as the *Stop, Observe, Breathe, Expand, Respond (SOBER) Breathing Space* can be effective (Witkiewitz et al., 2014). This practice involves pausing when a trigger arises, observing the situation mindfully, focusing on breathing, expanding awareness to encompass the whole body, and responding thoughtfully rather than impulsively.

Maintaining balance post-detox is undoubtedly challenging, but with structured approaches, it becomes manageable. Mindful practices enhance self-awareness, helping you stay attuned to your thoughts and feelings. Identifying and addressing triggers prevents potential setbacks, while regular goal setting and continuous progress evaluation sustain motivation and growth.

Dealing With Setbacks and Maintaining Vigilance

Handling setbacks effectively is pivotal for maintaining balance post-detox. By understanding how to navigate these challenges, you can remain devoted to your journey toward lasting change and avoid relapse after completing *The 21-day Dopamine Reset*.

Use Mistakes as Learning Curves

Setbacks are a natural part of any recovery journey. Rather than viewing them as failures, it's essential to see them as opportunities for learning and growth. When you experience a setback, take a step back and analyze what led to it. Was it a specific trigger, an environment, or a particular emotion? Identifying these factors can provide valuable insights into your behavior and help you develop strategies to prevent similar issues in the future.

For instance, if scrolling through social media late at night led to a relapse into old habits, recognize this pattern and adjust your routine. Perhaps, setting a curfew for device usage or finding alternative activities before bed could mitigate the issue. Embracing mistakes without self-blame encourages a proactive approach to personal growth and helps build a stronger foundation for continued progress.

Implementing Coping Strategies

Developing effective coping strategies is crucial for managing cravings and avoiding relapse triggers. Engaging in practices such as controlled breathing techniques, focused meditation, and progressive muscle relaxation can be exceptionally beneficial. These methods not only alleviate anxiety but also help shift attention away from desires for substances.

Identify your specific triggers, and devise personalized coping mechanisms for mitigating their impact. For example, if boredom often leads to unhealthy habits, create a list of engaging activities, such as reading, exercising, or creative hobbies, to keep yourself occupied. Having a few go-to coping strategies ensures that you have tools readily available when faced with challenging situations.

Staying Present

Practicing mindfulness is an effective way to stay focused on the present moment. Mindfulness involves being fully aware of your thoughts, feelings, and surroundings without judgment. This practice can help you become more attuned to your body's signals and your emotional state, making it easier to recognize early signs of stress or potential triggers.

Mindfulness can also enhance your appreciation for simple pleasures and reduce the urge to seek instant gratification through unhealthy means. By mindfully engaging in activities like walking, eating, or even doing household chores, they can be transformed into moments of calm and clarity.

Furthermore, mindfulness helps break the cycle of ruminative thinking, which often intensifies stress and anxiety. By maintaining focus on the present moment, you empower yourself to make intentional decisions that support your long-term aspirations, rather than succumbing to hasty reactions driven by short-term impulses.

Integrate brief mindfulness practices into your everyday life. Begin with five minutes of deep breathing in the morning or at night, and gradually extend the time as you grow more at ease with this technique.

Building Resilience

Resilience is the capacity to recover quickly from difficulties. You can build your resilience by transforming your negative thoughts into positive affirmations. For example, instead of thinking, *I can't handle this*, remind yourself, *I am capable of dealing with challenges*. Positive self-talk can shift your perspective and empower you to face obstacles with greater confidence.

Engaging in regular physical activity also bolsters resilience. Exercise has been proven to reduce symptoms of depression and anxiety, improve mood, and increase overall well-being. Whether it's a brisk walk, a yoga session, or a workout at the gym, incorporating physical activity into your routine can boost your mental strength.

Learning From Life's Challenges

Applying these principles to real-life scenarios can further enhance your resilience. Consider journaling about past experiences where you successfully overcame obstacles. Reflect on the strategies you used and how they contributed to your success. This reflection not only reinforces your capabilities but also serves as a reminder of your resilience during tough times.

Continuous learning and self-improvement play significant roles in building resilience. Enrolling in a new course, picking up a hobby, or even reading self-help books can equip you with additional skills and knowledge to tackle future challenges head-on.

Long-Term Strategies for Balanced Living

To support your goal of maintaining a healthy dopamine balance post-detox, integrating strategies and practices that promote ongoing well-being into your lifestyle is vital. Let's explore various approaches that can help you maintain a balanced approach to life beyond the initial detox period.

Prioritizing Self-Care

Self-care is fundamental to maintaining balance and nurturing holistic health. Incorporating self-care routines can significantly improve your physical, emotional, and mental well-being in the long term. For example, engaging in regular exercise that you enjoy is an excellent way to boost endorphins, which can elevate mood and reduce stress levels without relying on dopamine-spiking activities. Practicing physical activities you have fun doing is, therefore, a self-care practice that showcases your love for your mind and body.

Getting enough sleep is another critical aspect of self-care. Establishing a consistent sleep schedule and creating a relaxing bedtime routine—such as drinking herbal tea or reading a good book—can enhance sleep quality. Adequate sleep ensures that you wake up refreshed and ready to tackle the day's challenges.

Engaging in hobbies is also a form of self-care. Whether it's painting, gardening, or playing a musical instrument, pursuing interests outside of work enhances overall satisfaction and provides a necessary escape from the demands of everyday life. By prioritizing these self-care activities, you create a solid routine that helps you overcome the challenges of resisting a tempting lifestyle.

Exploring New Activities

The importance of engaging in new activities and hobbies can't be emphasized enough. Exploring new hobbies or interests after your detox can reinvigorate your sense of purpose and keep you mentally stimulated.

If you are a free and imaginative spirit, consider taking up a creative hobby like photography, painting, or writing. Creative pursuits can offer a therapeutic outlet for expressing emotions and thoughts. Additionally, they provide a sense of accomplishment and joy when you complete a project or improve a skill.

If you love to get your body moving, physical activities such as hiking, dancing, or joining a sports team can also be rewarding. Not only do they contribute to physical fitness, but they also offer opportunities to meet new people and build social connections. It's a win-win situation!

Learning a new language or instrument can also be intellectually stimulating. These activities challenge the brain, keeping it sharp and engaged. They require discipline and practice, which can translate into other areas of life, building your resilience and promoting a structured routine and persistence. There are so many new activities out there to try. Get out of your comfort zone by choosing something different that ignites a new passion within you.

Establishing Boundaries

Setting boundaries is essential for protecting yourself against potential triggers or overstimulation. Clear boundaries help maintain a balance after detox by ensuring that you have time and energy for self-care and personal interests.

Begin by identifying areas where boundaries are necessary. This might include limiting screen time, setting specific times for work and relaxation, or deciding how much—or what type of—social interaction you can handle without feeling overwhelmed. Communicate these boundaries clearly to others to avoid misunderstandings and ensure they respect your limits.

Consistency is key when enforcing boundaries. Once set, adhere to them diligently. For example, if you decide not to check work emails after 7 p.m., stick to this rule daily. Consistency reinforces the importance of these boundaries and makes it easier for others (and you) to respect them.

Make sure to prioritize self-care within your boundaries. Allocate time each day for activities that nurture your well-being, whether it's a morning workout, reading a book, or spending time by yourself to recharge. Ensuring self-care is part of your boundaries helps prevent burnout and maintains overall balance.

Seeking Professional Support

Considering professional support is crucial for ongoing guidance and support, especially after completing a detox. Therapy or counseling doesn't have to be reserved for your detox process, so don't be afraid to use the resources accessible to you indefinitely.

Therapists can offer tailored strategies to manage stress, cope with cravings, and address any underlying issues that may contribute to relapse. Regular therapy sessions create a safe space to discuss progress, setbacks, and goals, ensuring continuous personal growth and mental well-being (Perry, 2022).

Additionally, coaching services can help create personalized self-care plans that integrate seamlessly into your lifestyle. Coaches can assist in identifying effective self-care practices and establishing routines that promote work-life balance, further supporting long-term well-being (*Balancing Self-Care While Supporting...*, 2024).

Educational resources—such as books, online articles, and workshops—can supplement professional support. Thankfully, with this book in hand, you've already taken a huge first step in this regard. Educating yourself about maintaining balance and recognizing triggers equips you with the knowledge to make informed decisions and avoid pitfalls. Understanding different coping mechanisms and treatment options broadens your toolkit, enhancing your ability to maintain a healthy lifestyle suitable to you.

Recapping Maintenance Strategies for Post-Detox Success

This chapter has emphasized the importance of consistent monitoring and reflection to maintain lasting change after completing *The 21-day Dopamine Reset*. Establishing regular check-ins, utilizing habit-tracking tools, and seeking accountability from your support system and your personal routine are crucial strategies for preventing relapse and sustaining new habits. By scheduling regular reflection sessions, you can assess your progress, identify triggers, and set achievable short-term and long-term goals. Implementing these practices consistently helps reinforce positive behaviors and keeps the journey toward better mental well-being on track.

Additionally, incorporating healthy self-rewards and celebrating milestones fosters a positive feedback loop that encourages adherence to new routines. By integrating these strategies into your daily life, you can create a sustainable path toward improved mental health and holistic happiness.

Many others have walked down this path and are currently reaping the rewards from their hard work on consistency. You can be the next success story. In the next chapter, we will be uncovering some success stories that can inspire and instill hope in you, even when you face those challenging obstacles.

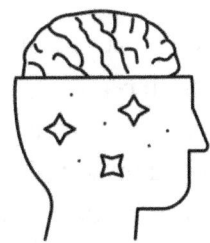

CHAPTER 10
Success Stories and Real-Life Applications

The millions of success stories and real-life applications of dopamine regulation that are out there illustrate the tangible benefits of structured detox plans. Individuals who have showcased perseverance and commitment to transforming their lives have witnessed a massive improvement in their lives, and their technology, food, and other behavioral addictions no longer have a hold on them. Reading through the stories of others can help you realize how possible it is for you to achieve this freedom from dopamine addiction as well.

This chapter delves into personal accounts of successful detox experiences, offering you actionable insights inspired by these narratives. By exploring how individuals before you navigated their detox journeys, you will discover effective strategies and valuable troubleshooting solutions. Additionally, we'll examine expert recommendations on dopamine regulation and habit formation, reinforcing the practical steps discussed in the personal stories. Through this blend of inspiration and practical advice, you will be equipped with the knowledge and motivation to embark on your own transformative detox journey.

Personal Accounts of Successful Detox Experiences

John Anderson's journey of resetting his dopamine levels and overcoming technology addiction is an inspiring story that showcases the transformative power of determination and commitment. John found himself spending countless hours on social media, gaming, and browsing the internet. This constant stimulation took a toll on his mental well-being, leading to decreased productivity, strained relationships, and a sense of dissatisfaction with life. He found himself so addicted to technology that he couldn't go an hour without scrolling through social media, watching TV, or having a digital device playing in the background.

Realizing the detrimental impact of his habits, John decided to embark on a detox journey. The first step he took was acknowledging his addiction and setting clear goals for his recovery. He began by scheduling specific times for using technology and gradually reducing those intervals. To reset his dopamine levels, John incorporated daily physical activities such as jogging and yoga, which helped him rewire his brain's reward system. He also started practicing mindfulness meditation to improve his focus and reduce stress.

Throughout this process, John faced numerous challenges, including withdrawal symptoms like irritability and anxiety. However, he persevered by reminding himself of his initial motivation and the positive changes he sought. One strategy that proved to be particularly effective was keeping a journal to track his progress. This allowed him to reflect on his achievements and setbacks and make necessary adjustments to his plan.

John's commitment to his detox plan yielded significant improvements in his life. He noticed increased mental clarity, better sleep quality, and enhanced relationships with family and friends. By limiting his screen time, John discovered new interests and hobbies, like painting and hiking, which further contributed to his overall well-being.

His story is a testament to the power of perseverance and the positive impact of implementing a structured detox plan in daily life.

Another remarkable success story is that of Sarah Jones, whose detox journey transformed her mental well-being. Sarah struggled with anxiety and depression, worsened by her excessive use of social media and constant exposure to negative news. Her addiction to technology also fostered a toxic relationship with food. She found herself in a routine of binge eating that started consuming her life and her overall health. Every time she felt anxious, she would turn to social media and food for emotional comfort. Determined to regain control over her life, she decided to undertake a detox program that focused on reducing her reliance on digital devices and improving her mental health.

Sarah started by identifying the sources of her stress and devising strategies to limit their influence. She set boundaries for her social media usage, such as disabling notifications and allocating specific times for checking updates. To fill the void left by reduced screen time, she engaged in activities that promoted relaxation and positivity, and she discovered just how much she enjoyed reading, gardening, and spending time with loved ones.

A crucial aspect of Sarah's success was the support system she built around her. She joined a local support group where members shared their experiences and encouraged one another throughout their detox journeys. This sense of community provided Sarah with the motivation and accountability she needed to stay committed to her goals. She also sought professional help from a therapist who guided her through cognitive behavioral techniques to manage her anxiety and develop healthier coping mechanisms.

As Sarah progressed in her detox journey, she experienced profound changes in her mental state. Her anxiety levels decreased, and she felt more in control of her emotions. The reduced exposure to negative news and social media drama allowed her to focus on the positive aspects of her life, fostering a sense of gratitude and contentment. She also healed her relationship with food. She ate to nourish her body and spoiled herself with treats when she felt like it, instead of resorting to binge eating for a sense of emotional relief. Sarah's experience highlights the importance of a supportive environment and the role it plays in achieving successful detox outcomes.

Both John and Sarah's stories illustrate the transformative potential of a well-structured detox plan. Their journeys emphasize the importance of commitment, perseverance, and support systems in overcoming addictive behaviors and improving mental well-being. By learning about all the different real-life examples out there, you can draw inspiration and motivation to embark on your own detox journey.

One key lesson from John's experience is the significance of setting clear goals and tracking progress. As we have learned, keeping a journal not only helps in monitoring achievements but also provides a sense of accomplishment and motivation. This strategy can be incredibly beneficial for anyone trying to break free from technology addiction or other unhealthy habits.

Sarah's journey, on the other hand, emphasizes the critical role of support systems. Whether it's joining a local group or seeking professional help, having a network of people who understand and encourage your efforts can make a substantial difference. The sense of community and shared experiences can provide the necessary boost to maintain commitment and overcome challenges.

Implementing specific strategies to overcome obstacles is another valuable takeaway from these stories. Both John and Sarah devised practical approaches tailored to their needs and circumstances. John incorporated physical activities and mindfulness practices to reset his dopamine levels, while Sarah focused on creating boundaries for her social media usage and engaging in relaxing activities. These personalized strategies highlight the importance of finding what works best for you and adapting your plan accordingly.

Expert Interviews and Testimonials

Expert perspectives and recommendations can further enhance your detox experience. Exploring the science behind dopamine regulation and habit formation provides a foundational understanding of how our brains react to various stimuli. Dr. Luisa Speranza, a renowned neuroscientist, sheds light on this subject to further help you comprehend why certain habits form and how they can be reprogrammed.

As you know, dopamine is a neurotransmitter that is often associated with feelings of pleasure and reward, and it plays a crucial role in habit formation. The mesolimbic pathway, also known as the "reward system," governs our response to rewarding stimuli. When engaging in activities that spike dopamine levels, the brain essentially "rewires" itself, reinforcing these behaviors and making them more likely to be repeated. Dr. Speranza explains that understanding this mechanism allows you to identify triggers and implement strategies better suited for your personal detox journey. For example, gradually reducing your exposure to high-dopamine triggers can help mitigate withdrawal symptoms and ease the transition to healthier habits by increasing neuroplasticity—the brain's ability to reshape itself in response to new stimuli (Speranza et al., 2021).

Dr. Ryan R. Bailey, a behavioral psychiatrist, offers insights into maintaining habit sustainability and modifying behaviors effectively. According to Dr. Bailey, the key lies in setting realistic goals and employing consistent reinforcement methods. She emphasizes the importance of small, incremental changes rather than drastic, overwhelming shifts. This approach ensures that new habits are manageable, helping to bridge what is known as the "intention-behavior gap" (Bailey, 2017). Incorporating self-monitoring practices, like journaling progress and setbacks, helps maintain accountability and provides valuable feedback for continuous improvement.

Coping with triggers that may initiate a relapse requires strategic planning and can be aided by professional advice. Recognizing potential triggers—whether emotional, environmental, or social—is the first step. Once identified, creating an action plan to address these triggers becomes essential. For instance, if stress at work tends to lead to unhealthy habits, developing healthy work-life boundaries and alternative stress-relief techniques—such as mindfulness meditation, exercise, or creative hobbies—can serve as both prevention and treatment of this trigger.

Notably, access to pharmacological aids can also come into play, as highlighted by Espinosa-Salas & Gonzalez-Arias (2023). They state that medications like bupropion and varenicline have been effective in smoking cessation by targeting specific neurotransmitter pathways. While these options are not the primary focus of most detox plans aimed at breaking digital or non-substance-related habits, they illustrate how comprehensive approaches that encompass both behavioral and pharmacological strategies can enhance overall outcomes.

In a corporate environment saturated with digital stimuli and high-stress demands, a dopamine reset program can be transformative. For many people, detoxing involves periods of abstaining from dopamine-stimulating activities such as social media, excessive caffeine consumption, and compulsive checking of emails. This intentional break allows employees to recalibrate their reward systems and ultimately boosts productivity and personal well-being.

Thankfully, the need for dopamine regulation is becoming more and more recognized, even in the corporate world. For instance, the tech company Innovate Hub implemented a 30-day dopamine reset challenge for its employees. Participants were guided to limit their exposure to digital distractions and instead engage in mindfulness practices like meditation and yoga. Initial feedback revealed that employees felt more focused and less overwhelmed. Over time, many reported improved mental clarity and creativity. These positive outcomes underscore the potential benefits of incorporating dopamine reset programs into corporate wellness initiatives.

Organizational support plays a crucial role in the success of such interventions. When management endorses and encourages these programs, it sends a strong message about the organization's commitment to employee health and happiness. Innovate Hub's leadership provided scheduled breaks for mindfulness activities and established no-email periods during certain hours. This collective approach not only bolstered individual efforts but also fostered a culture of mutual accountability and support, which significantly enhanced adherence to the program and expanded its benefits across the team.

However, even in a group scenario such as this, the journey of transformation through a dopamine detox program can be deeply personal and profound. Take the case of Emily, a marketing executive who had battled with technology addiction: Her typical day was consumed by endless scrolling through social media, checking work emails incessantly, and filling her downtime with online shopping. Recognizing the need for change, she embarked on a six-week dopamine detox. Though it was initially challenging, Emily gradually reduced her out-of-work screen time, replacing it with healthier activities like reading, cooking, and spending quality time with friends and family.

Emily's step-by-step progress was marked by several phases. In the first week, she struggled with withdrawal symptoms such as irritability and restlessness, but she remained committed. By the second week, she noticed an improvement in her sleep patterns and a reduction in her anxiety levels. Midway through the program, Emily began experiencing natural highs from non-digital activities. By the end of the six weeks, Emily felt rejuvenated and more present in her daily life.

What's more, the ripple effects of the lifestyle changes brought on by a dopamine detox extend beyond the individual. Emily's improved mental state also positively impacted her relationships. She became more engaged during family dinners and more attentive to her children's needs. This shift did not go unnoticed; her spouse remarked on how much happier and more connected the entire family felt. On a broader scale, Emily's newfound balance and tranquility translated to higher productivity at work, leading to better performance and job satisfaction. Her colleagues observed her transformation, inspiring several to embark on their own detox journeys.

Understanding the science behind these interventions further solidifies their rationale. Dopamine can become dysregulated with constant stimulation. Dr. Amanda Lee emphasizes the importance of structured breaks to reset these pathways and restore motivation. Abstinence from overstimulation is pivotal, but equally important are the activities chosen to replace unhelpful habits. By integrating practices that elevate mood naturally—such as exercise, mindfulness, and social interactions—the detox process becomes more effective and sustainable (Fuchs, 2022).

Relapse prevention is another critical component for lasting change. Strategies to combat relapse include setting clear boundaries and finding healthy replacements for dopamine-spiking activities. For example, if social media was the primary source of dopamine spikes, substituting it with engaging non-digital hobbies like gardening or painting can provide fulfilling alternatives. Regular check-ins with a support system—whether through friends, family, or professional counseling—can offer ongoing encouragement and accountability.

Behavioral psychologists like Dr. Alex Carter highlight the complexities of addiction and stress the importance of supervised interventions. Professional support ensures that you understand the underlying mechanisms of dopamine regulation and receive personalized strategies suited to your unique circumstances. This tailored approach minimizes risks associated with withdrawal and maximizes the probability of long-term success.

It's valuable to know how we can learn from others and use their experiences as a roadmap for our own success. None of us have to live life all on our own. We can teach and guide each other, preventing the same mistakes. Joining supportive networks doesn't just offer you a space to communicate your frustrations freely; it also provides you with a variety of personal stories you can use to make informed decisions throughout your journey.

In this chapter, we explored the transformative power of sharing personal success stories and practical strategies for overcoming technology addiction and improving your lifestyle. Through John Anderson and Sarah Jones's journeys, we've learned the importance of commitment, setting clear goals, and building a supportive environment. Their experiences highlight how structured detox plans, physical activities, mindfulness practices, and professional guidance can lead to significant improvements in life quality, mental clarity, and relationships.

By examining expert insights and real-life examples, we have gained valuable knowledge on resetting our dopamine levels, managing relapses, and sustaining positive habits. The diverse interventions discussed serve as a toolkit for you as you embark on your own detox journey. Through gradual changes, personalized strategies, and resilient coping mechanisms, anyone can take steps towards a healthier, more fulfilling lifestyle. Let your story be the next success by making changes in your habits and routine that can transform your life as you know it!

CONCLUSION

After a journey of learning and practicing dopamine detox activities, let's take a moment to pause and reflect on what you've achieved over the past 21 days or what you've discovered before embarking on this turbulent adventure. This is more than a mere detox; it is a meaningful exploration into your habits, behaviors, and ways of thinking. At its core, this journey is about understanding the profound impact of dopamine and how it shapes your daily life. By recognizing the power of this neurotransmitter, you have taken significant steps toward reducing overstimulation and reclaiming control over your mental well-being.

Throughout these three weeks, we delved into the concept of dopamine and its role in forming habits; we explored how our constant exposure to technology can overwhelm our brains, leading to stress, anxiety, and a diminished capacity for joy. You learned practical strategies for disconnecting from dopamine-spiking activities, setting boundaries, and finding healthier, more fulfilling activities to replace those that no longer serve you.

Our modern lives are inundated with stimuli, from the endless scroll of social media to the relentless ping of notifications. These sources of overstimulation can hijack your brain's reward system, leaving you perpetually seeking the next hit of dopamine. In this book, you've discovered that taking a step back—detoxifying your mind—is not about deprivation but rather making room for the things that truly matter: deep connections, meaningful experiences, and genuine well-being.

The first critical lesson is the undeniable influence of dopamine on your habits. Becoming aware of this influence gives you the ability to make conscious choices. For example, you may now realize that craving another episode of a TV show or endlessly scrolling through your phone is not a result of a lack of willpower but a response to dopamine-driven habits formed over time. This awareness is empowering because it means you can change these patterns by introducing new, healthier habits that provide lasting fulfillment.

The importance of reducing overstimulation is crucial because our brains were not designed to handle the barrage of information and sensory input that modern technology provides. By intentionally creating space in your life—whether through mindfulness practices, spending time in nature, or simply enjoying quiet moments—you are giving your brain the chance to recover and recalibrate.

As you move beyond the structured 21-day plan, it's crucial to recognize that the journey does not end here. The changes you've implemented are not short-term fixes but foundational shifts toward a more balanced and mindful way of living. The strategies you have practiced—mindful tech usage, establishing boundaries, and engaging in rewarding offline activities—are tools you can continue to refine and adapt as you move forward.

Consider the long-term benefits of sustaining these healthy habits. Continuing to practice mindfulness, regularly checking in with yourself, and engaging in physical activity are all ways to maintain and even deepen the positive changes you've initiated. Think about how these habits have already started to improve your life. Maybe, you feel less anxious, more in control, or better able to focus on meaningful tasks. These are stepping stones to a more fulfilling life.

For a moment, take the opportunity to reflect deeply on your personal growth over the past few weeks. What challenges did you encounter, and how did you overcome them? Perhaps, there were moments when you slipped back into old habits or found it difficult to resist the pull of high-dopamine activities or substances. Acknowledge these moments not as failures but as valuable learning experiences. Each challenge faced and each small victory achieved has contributed to your resilience and self-awareness.

Think about the ways in which you've grown. Maybe, you've discovered a new hobby that brings you joy, reconnected with loved ones on a deeper level, or simply found peace in moments of stillness. These are significant milestones worth celebrating. Your commitment to breaking free from unhealthy habits is commendable, and every step you've taken has brought you closer to becoming the best version of yourself.

Personal growth takes time and consistent effort, so be patient with yourself. There will always be new challenges and opportunities to learn. Embrace these moments with the same curiosity and determination that brought you this far. By reflecting on your progress regularly, you ensure that the positive changes you've made become firmly embedded in your daily life.

As you conclude this book, let's look ahead with optimism and intention. The path to a balanced life is ongoing, and maintaining the progress you've made requires continuous effort and dedication. Prioritize your well-being, make mindfulness a daily practice, and cultivate habits that foster mental and emotional health.

Your journey does not end with this book; it continues each day. Commit to nurturing yourself, cherishing meaningful connections, and pursuing activities that bring you true satisfaction. Remember that balance is not a final destination but a state of being that you can strive for every day. Continue to seek harmony in your interactions with technology and the world around you. Pursuing a balanced life will undoubtedly bring you closer to the enriched and harmonious future you deserve!

Thank you for reading! If you enjoyed this book, please take a moment to leave a quick star rating for this author, and don't forget to check out the full library of interesting topics available in this author's library of work.

REFERENCES

Achieving sobriety with SMART goals for opiod use disorder. (2024, March 11). Waterstone Counseling Centers. https://waterstonecenter.com/achieving-sobriety-with-smart-goals-for-opioid-use-disorder/

Addiction Blog. (n.d.). Practical Recovery. https://www.practicalrecovery.com/practical-recovery-blog/

Al-Thaqib, A., Al-Sultan, F., Al-Zahrani, A., Al-Kahtani, F., Al-Regaiey, K., Iqbal, M., & Bashir, S. (2018). Brain training games enhance cognitive function in healthy subjects. *Medical Science Monitor Basic Research*, 20(24), 63-69. https://doi.org/10.12659/msmbr.909022

Bailey, R.R. (2017). Goal setting and action planning for health behavior change. *American Journal of Lifestyle Medicine*, 13(6), 615–618. https://doi.org/10.1177/1559827617729634

Balancing self-care while supporting an addicted loved one. (2024, July 17). Harmony Ridge Recovery Center. https://www.harmonyridgerecovery.com/balancing-self-care-supporting-addicted-loved-one/

BookAuthority. (2024). *20 best food addiction books of all time.* Lifehack Labs. https://bookauthority.org/books/best-food-addiction-books

Bromberg-Martin, E. S., Matsumoto, M., & Hikosaka, O. (2010, December 9). Dopamine in motivational control: Rewarding, aversive, and alerting. *Neuron*, 68(5), 815–834. https://doi.org/10.1016/j.neuron.2010.11.022

Chowdhury, M. R. (2019, April 9). *The neuroscience of gratitude and effects on the brain.* PositivePsychology. https://positivepsychology.com/neuroscience-of-gratitude/

Cleveland Clinic. (2023, March 16). *Addiction.* https://my.clevelandclinic.org/health/diseases/6407-addiction

Daily rituals to boost health and happiness. (n.d.). Nivati. https://www.nivati.com/blog/daily-rituals-to-boost-health-and-happiness

Daily routine: Digital detox: Digital detox: Reclaiming your life from technology in your daily routine. (n.d.). FasterCapital. https://fastercapital.com/content/Daily-Routine--Digital-Detox--Digital-Detox--Reclaiming-Your-Life-from-Technology-in-Your-Daily-Routine.html

Dealing with setbacks in recovery. (2023, June 23). Anchored Tides Recovery. https://anchoredtidesrecovery.com/dealing-with-setbacks-in-recovery/

Delaney, E. (2023, August 16). *What is the dopamine diet?* BBC Good Food. https://www.bbcgoodfood.com/howto/guide/what-dopamine-diet

Dellwo, A. (2023, April 17). *Dopamine: What it does for you and related conditions.* Verywell Health. https://www.verywellhealth.com/dopamine-5086831

Digital detox 101: Reclaim your peace and productivity. (2024, July 30). Heal.me. https://heal.me/articles/digital-detox-101-reclaim-your-peace-and-productivity

Digital detox – the best tips for a digital time-out. (2024, June 10). OVB. https://www.ovb.eu/english/blog/article/digital-detox-the-best-tips-for-a-digital-time-out.html

Dopamine fasting probably doesn't work, try this instead. (2019, November 13). Psych Central. https://psychcentral.com/blog/dopamine-fasting-probably-doesnt-work-try-this-instead

Dresp-Langley, B. (2023, September 1). From reward to anhedonia - Dopamine function in the global mental health context. *Biomedicines*, 11(9), 2469. https://doi.org/10.3390/biomedicines11092469

Ducci, F., & Goldman, D. (2012, June). The genetic basis of addictive disorders. *Psychiatric Clinics of North America*, 35(2), 495–519. https://doi.org/10.1016/j.psc.2012.03.010

Eatontown, D. P. R. (2022, October 14). *5 healthy & unhealthy coping skills.* Positive Reset Mental Health Services of Eatontown New Jersey. https://positivereseteatontown.com/5-healthy-unhealthy-coping-skills/

Espinosa-Salas, S., & Gonzalez-Arias, M. (2023). *Behavior modification for lifestyle improvement.* PubMed; StatPearls Publishing. https://www.ncbi.nlm.nih.gov/books/NBK592418/

5 Tips to Help You Stick to Your Recovery Goals. (2024, May 14). All Points North. https://apn.com/resources/5-tips-to-help-you-stick-to-your-recovery-goals/

Food addiction and the dopamine connection. (n.d.). Alchemy Cryotherapy Centre. https://alchemycryo.com.au/blog/food-addiction-and-the-dopamine-connection

Fuchs, M. (2022, March 7). *How to get healthier dopamine highs.* Time. https://time.com/6155109/healthier-dopamine-highs/

Fuente González, C. E., Chávez-Servín, J. L., de la Torre-Carbot, K., Ronquillo González, D., Aguilera Barreiro, M. de los Á., & Ojeda Navarro, L. R. (2022, May 18). Relationship between emotional eating, consumption of hyperpalatable energy-dense foods, and indicators of nutritional status: A systematic review. *Journal of Obesity*. https://doi.org/10.1155/2022/4243868

Gardner, E. L. (2011). Addiction and brain reward and antireward pathways. *Chronic Pain and Addiction*, 30, 22-60. https://doi.org/10.1159/000324065

Gunton, A. V. (2024, May 10). *Mindfulness based relapse prevention MBRP*. Recovered on Purpose. https://recoveredonpurpose.org/mindfulness-based-relapse-prevention/

How to bring meaningful rituals into your daily life. (n.d.). Calm Blog. https://www.calm.com/blog/how-to-bring-meaningful-rituals-into-your-daily-life

How to rebuild your life: Strategies for long-term recovery. (2024, May 29). Positive Recovery Centers. https://positiverecovery.com/how-to-rebuild-your-life-strategies-for-long-term-recovery/

Jimenez, R. (2023, December 13). *7-day digital detox challenge: The surprising health benefits you need to know*. Money Hacking Mama. https://moneyhackingmama.com/digital-detox-challenge/

Lewis, R. G., Florio, E., Punzo, D., & Borrelli, E. (2021). The brain's reward system in health and disease. *Advances in Experimental Medicine and Biology*, 1344, 57–69. https://doi.org/10.1007/978-3-030-81147-1_4

Looney, S. (2022, March 31). *The importance of small wins*. Sonya Looney. https://sonyalooney.com/the-importance-of-small-wins/

Lorenz, K. (2019, December 5). *Screen addiction affects physical and mental health*. Premier Health. https://www.premierhealth.com/your-health/articles/health-topics/screen-addiction-affects-physical-and-mental-health

Kletzel, S. L., Sood, P., Negm, A., Heyn, P. C., Krishnan, S., Machtinger, J., Hu, X., & Devos, H. (2021, June). Effectiveness of brain gaming in older adults with cognitive impairments: A systematic review and meta-analysis. *Journal of the American*

Medical Directors Association, 22(11), 2281–2288. https://doi.org/10.1016/j.jamda.2021.05.022

Maladaptive coping: Understanding and overcoming harmful strategies. (n.d.). SonderMind. https://www.sondermind.com/resources/articles-and-content/maladaptive-coping/

Mandocdoc, M. (2024, February 19). *Recovery - Navigating setbacks: Five strategies for resilience.* Kolmac Integrated Behavioral Health Centers. https://www.kolmac.com/navigating-setbacks-on-your-substance-use-recovery-journey-five-strategies-for-resilience/

Martino, J., Pegg, J., & Frates, E. P. (2017, October 7). The connection prescription: Using the power of social interactions and the deep desire for connectedness to empower health and wellness. *American Journal of Lifestyle Medicine*, 11(6), 466–475. https://doi.org/10.1177/1559827615608788

Miller, K. (2019, July 4). *5 ways to develop a growth mindset: Start building your grit and resilience today.* PositivePsychology. https://positivepsychology.com/5-ways-develop-grit-resilience/

Mindfulness practices for managing addiction and health. (2024, February 28). Your Health Magazine. https://yourhealthmagazine.net/article/addiction/mindfulness-practices-for-managing-addiction-and-health/

Nakshine, V. S., Thute, P., Khatib, M. N., & Sarkar, B. (2022, October 8). *Increased screen time as a cause of declining physical, psychological health, and sleep patterns: A literary review.* Cureus. https://www.cureus.com/articles/112862-increased-screen-time-as-a-cause-of-declining-physical-psychological-health-and-sleep-patterns-a-literary-review

National Center for Complementary and Integrative Health. (2022, June). *Meditation and mindfulness: What you need to know.*

https://www.nccih.nih.gov/health/meditation-and-mindfulness-what-you-need-to-know

National Institute on Drug Abuse. (2023, March 22). *New NIH study reveals shared genetic markers underlying substance use disorders.* https://nida.nih.gov/news-events/news-releases/2023/03/new-nih-study-reveals-shared-genetic-markers-underlying-substance-use-disorders

National Institute on Drug Abuse. (2020). *Drugs and the Brain.* https://nida.nih.gov/publications/drugs-brains-behavior-science-addiction/drugs-brain

9 fast, easy ways to boost dopamine (the doing/motivation hormone). (2023, April 12). Bethany Medical Clinic. https://www.bmcofny.com/9-fast-easy-ways-to-boost-dopamine-the-doing-motivation-hormone/

Northwestern Medicine. (2022, November 1). *The role of dopamine in habit formation and compulsive behavior with Talia Lerner, PhD.* Feinberg School of Medicine. https://www.feinberg.northwestern.edu/research/podcast/2022/role-of-dopamine-habit-formation-talia-lerner%20.html

100 suggested habits to track in your habit calendar. (n.d.). Free Period Press. https://freeperiodpress.com/blogs/free-period-press-blog/100-suggested-habits-to-track

Perry, E. (2022, September 10). *Self-care and work-life balance: How to take care of yourself.* BetterUp. https://www.betterup.com/blog/self-care-and-work-life-balance

10 hobbies to explore at rehab. (2024, March, 25). Harmony Ridge Recovery Center. https://www.harmonyridgerecovery.com/10-hobbies-to-explore-at-rehab/

The power of a digital detox (Episode #746) [Audio podcast]. (2022, December 29). Solluna With Kimberly Snyder. https://mysolluna.com/blog/the-power-of-a-digital-detox-episode-746/

The power of mindful self-compassion for personal growth. (2024, March 26). MindShift Zone. https://mindshift.zone/blog/the-power-of-mindful-self-compassion-for-personal-growth/

Preventing relapse: Advice for keeping yourself accountable. (2024, June 17). Valley Hospital. https://valleyhospital-phoenix.com/uncategorized/preventing-relapse-advice-for-keeping-yourself-accountable/

Russell, M. (2024, May 30). *Why celebrating small wins matters.* Harvard Summer School. https://summer.harvard.edu/blog/why-celebrating-small-wins-matters/

Schuman-Olivier, Z., Trombka, M., Lovas, D. A., Brewer, J. A., Vago, D. R., Gawande, R., Dunne, J. P., Lazar, S. W., Loucks, E. B., & Fulwiler, C. (2020). Mindfulness and behavior change. *Harvard Review of Psychiatry*, 28(6), 371–395. https://doi.org/10.1097/HRP.0000000000000277

Signs and symptoms of addiction. (n.d.). Psychology Today. https://www.psychologytoday.com/us/basics/addiction/signs-and-symptoms-addiction

Speranza, L., di Porzio, U., Viggiano, D., de Donato, A. & Volpicelli, F. (2021). Dopamine: The neuromodulator of long-term synaptic plasticity, reward and movement control. *Cells*, 10(4), 735. https://doi.org/10.3390/cells10040735

Sutter Health. (2019). *Eating well for mental health.* https://www.sutterhealth.org/health/nutrition/eating-well-for-mental-health

Travers, M. (n.d.). *A psychologist explains the neuroscience of your "gratitude practice."* Forbes. https://www.forbes.com/sites/traversmark/2024/05/22/a-psychologist-explains-how-to-hack-your-brains-gratitude-circuit/

23 Apps That Will Keep You Accountable. (2023). Goals Won. https://www.goalswon.com/blog/23-apps-that-will-keep-you-accountable-and-motivated-to-achieve-all-your-personal-goals

UC Davis Health. (2022, December 14). *10 health benefits of meditation and how to focus on mindfulness.* Cultivating Health. https://health.ucdavis.edu/blog/cultivating-health/10-health-benefits-of-meditation-and-how-to-focus-on-mindfulness-and-compassion/2022/12

Umberson, D., & Karas Montez, J. (2010, August 4). Social relationships and health: A flashpoint for health policy. *Journal of Health and Social Behavior,* 51(1), 54–66. https://doi.org/10.1177/0022146510383501

Vyas, N. (2023, July 18). *How lack of sleep impacts cognitive performance and focus.* Sleep Foundation. https://www.sleepfoundation.org/sleep-deprivation/lack-of-sleep-and-cognitive-impairment

Walker, D. J. (2024, April 10). *What's on your plate? How healthy eating can fuel your mental health.* TimelyCare. https://timelycare.com/blog/whats-on-your-plate-how-healthy-eating-can-fuel-your-mental-health/

Ufot, R. S. (2023, August 31). *Digital detox: Journey to freedom from digital chains.* Medium. https://medium.com/@rebeccausunday/digital-detox-journey-to-freedom-from-digital-chains-c77aa2441d15

Watson, S. (2021, July 20). *Dopamine: The pathway to pleasure.* Harvard Health; Harvard Medical School. https://www.health.harvard.edu/mind-and-mood/dopamine-the-pathway-to-pleasure

Wein, H. (2021, March 29). *Good sleep for good health.* NIH News in Health; National Institutes of Health. https://newsinhealth.nih.gov/2021/04/good-sleep-good-health

Wise, R. A., & Jordan, C. J. (2021). Dopamine, behavior, and addiction. *Journal of Biomedical Science*, 28(1), 83. https://doi.org/10.1186/s12929-021-00779-7

Witkiewitz, K., Bowen, S., Harrop, E. N., Douglas, H., Enkema, M., &; Sedgwick, C. (2014, March 11). Mindfulness-based treatment to prevent addictive behavior relapse: Theoretical models and hypothesized mechanisms of change. *Substance Use & Misuse*, 49(5), 513–524. https://doi.org/10.3109/10826084.2014.891845

Yau, Y. H. C., & Potenza, M. N. (2013, September). *Stress and eating behaviors.* Minerva Endocrinologica, 38(3), 255–267. https://www.ncbi.nlm.nih.gov/pmc/articles/PMC4214609/

www.ingramcontent.com/pod-product-compliance
Lightning Source LLC
Chambersburg PA
CBHW071032240526
45469CB00006BD/2184